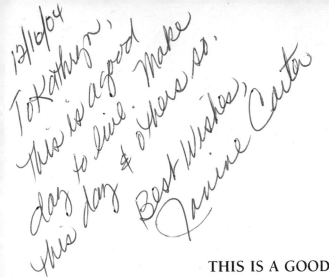

12/10/04
To Kathryn,
This is a good
day to live. Make
this day & others so.
Best Wishes,
Janine Carter

THIS IS A GOOD DAY TO LIVE

By
Janine Carter

The Library of Congress has catalogued this edition as follows:
Carter, Janine
This is a Good Day to Live/by Janine Carter
ISBN 097631690

Introduction

This book is my sister's story of love, hope, pain, and life. It is a story of a young girl struggling every day with the dilemmas of college friends, family, and self-esteem. All that a normal teenager deals with, except hers was more complicated: She had cancer.

Now, as a mother of two beautiful boys, it has been my privilege to sit and read Amber's story, living it again through her eyes.

As you read this book, you will become a part of the family. You will know a mother's role as a caretaker of her first born baby. You will know a father's duty to try and fix it all and support his family financially. As her sister, too young to understand what is happening, you will see how I tried to cope. Also a teenager, I tried to find a way to deal with my big sister being sick.

You will know a courageous, young woman's positive attitude as she fights for her life day by day. My hope is that you will read Amber's story and know why we all must live each day to the fullest.

Bridgett Carter-Janowicz

Forward

Oncologists walk a line between getting close to patients at an emotional distance. If you get too close, loss takes a heavy toll. If you stay too far away you never get to appreciate the beauty of the person – their uniqueness, their life experiences. You miss out on the lessons that they can teach you – and your emotional connection is less sincere.

With Amber Carter, it was immediately clear that I would get close to her. She had the qualities that made it a certainty I would be touched by her. She had a sweetness that was completely natural, warm and attentive eyes and an appreciative supportive smile. She was trusting, intelligent and kind. And she had an unspoken confidence in me, which made me always try extra hard to do my best for her.

As you will learn in this book, Amber also was given the gift of a loving, caring family, and it is through the diaries of Amber, her mother and her sister that we are given an intimate personal view of their thoughts as they traveled the difficult journey of Amber's illness with her.

When I first met Amber and realized that we would be close, I imagined a happy story. I anticipated that the cancer would be cured, that I would attend Amber's college graduation, that I would dance at her wedding, and that I would remain in touch as she became a mother. I imagined that I would know and enjoy her children. But these expectations were met with disappointment. And as chronicled in the book, we never got past the first expectation. Her Hodgkin's lymphoma was not cured. In spite of chemotherapy, radiation, and ultimately a bone marrow transplant, the lymphoma was relentless and it took her life.

Stories about cancer, with examples of the courage of people who face this beast, always lead to questions about the meaning of life. This is another testament to the truth that life is about love. Life is given meaning by the giving and receiving of love.

Amber had an unlimited capacity to give love and as a result she received boundless love from those whose lives she touched. Her short life had rich meaning. She gave and received love. I will always treasure my memory of her and this book will allow you to know her also.

Daniel R. Lewis, M.D.

Preface

Amber,

You came to me with fear and your own yearning to stay and live longer—to be well again.

Together we practiced living this one moment, shifting in and out of pain, frustration, sadness, joy, and laughter. You shared yourself in the deepest, purest ways, with talk, and art and clay.

You shed your tears because you felt you burdened and disappointed your beloved family when test results were bad. You worried for their well-being. You loved your grandmother and your time with her in the house by the river. You talked of the big tree with its low swooping branches where you played house with Bridgett in Albuquerque. You remembered health.

You reached through the unfairness of it all to something deeper. You knew the urgency at times and we repeated the prayers of acceptance:

This is a good day to live

This is a good day to die

This is a good day

You told me it brought you peace.

I will miss my Fridays with you, Amber. I will miss your pure Spirit reborn to a Pure Land.

Roslyn Strohl, MFT

This book is dedicated to all those who "fought the good fight" especially

Elena Nicole Macedo
March 15, 1990 – September 2, 1998

Erin Rebecca Johnson
April 17, 1978 – June 17, 1996

Amber Leahanne Carter
August 8 1976 – June 10 1999

To my family, Tom and Bridgett, who never faltered in the hope for this book, and consistently believed I could finish it, even when I thought I couldn't. To my dear mother, Verna Castleman, the wind beneath my wings, who died before this book could become a reality.

Author's Notes

In my effort to organize my thoughts on paper taken from my personal journals, I found it necessary to edit my language and polish my grammar. As are most intimate journals/diaries, the important factor in formulating the written word is just to get it down on paper while the feelings are fresh. Because I can, I have re-written these thoughts, based on the facts as I remembered them in these daily writings.

This is not the case with the journals of my sweet Amber. Her written word is pure with the exception of any additional explanations necessary for clarity of thought. These changes are noted within the text by ( ) surrounding any word or sentence. In the instance of a misspelled word, I have left it intact to show the maturity level and simple thought process she had while writing her tender and sometimes injured feelings.

The journal entries of Bridgett have been left intact and with her permission without benefit of correction of spelling and grammar. If they are altered it is because she wished it so.

In order to show the different voices of the three of us, the following rules apply:

a) I have chosen to put my own words in regular Berkley Book font.

b) *Amber's voice is indicated in the same font, only italicized.*

c) Bridgett's writing is in Berkley Medium, and signed at the end with her initials, BC.

d) Unless otherwise noted, all poetry is by Janine Carter.

Release of Liability

I have taken my daily journal writings and used them accordingly as reference material. The many medical terms used are from my recollection. Procedures, treatments, names of drugs, alternative medicines, and methods are used through out this book and in no way are meant to suggest their usage as one preferred method over another.

I do not pretend to be anything but a faithfully involved mother of a daughter who had cancer. The opinions given here are by me and only are based on fact and written in my words. Names have been altered to avoid any misconception on the part of those who interacted with our family during the last five years of Amber's precious life. If real names have been used it is with their permission.

In Gratitude

Each day I read a few daily books of affirmations. A year after Amber died, I looked at the entry in one of them for June 10th. It reads:

"The greatest gift we can give is rapt attention to one another's existence. Of one thing we can be certain: we each are in this world by design. Further, we are in on another's daily travels by invitation. We share a destiny, and our understanding and joy will be proportionate to our sincere attention to those we're obviously accompanying.

No opportunity for an exchange of words, simple gestures, quiet thoughts should be discounted or denied. Each moment of our lives offers us the necessary experiences for our full potential. We need one another's presence, contributions, even tribulations in order to move forward together as well as individually."

I have not been able to locate this book since I copied this page five years ago and sent in a card to commemorate the one year anniversary of Amber's passing. I believe it was divinely sent. This is the way I feel about the people I have listed here. You were all there for our family when we needed you.

Verna and Larry Castleman
Dorothy and Bob Stueber
Joan and Don McGinnis
Camille and John Stueber
Janice and Bill Pollard
Judy and Joe Chiado
Eva and Joe Davalos
Amanda Chiado-Bozzi
Bridgett and Matt Janowicz
Debby Simms-Sagisi

All of "Amber's Angels"
        You know who you are
        God bless you all !

Suzanne Caplette-Champeau*

St. Patrick's parish members
        who prayed for Amber
Fr. Ron Shirley
Fr. Joseph Butters
Sr. Eva O'Dea
Sr. Regina Roche
Jay Horn
Holly Kelly
Sharon Brandy*
Cindy and Jim Fogarty

Dr. Daniel Lewis*
Ann "Red" Fontenou*
Ann Rempe
Faith Ann Fieldhouse
Linda Nowlen
Jan Shields
Evelyn Bovee

French Hospital Pediatrics
"Peds" Pati Merdinger
Rosie Cullen
 Lynne Lane
Dr. Tom Miller
Helen Rowan

Sierra Vista ambulatory
Aki Alimashrab
Sue Ann Allisandro
Dr. "Howie" Hayashi
Dr. Robert Stewart

Wellness Community Foothills
Angel Flights
Sisters of my 12 Step group
Ann Rock
Donna Covey
Grandma and Grandpa Rogers
          Lessie and Bill
Roseanne Seitz

City of Hope
Karen McCurdy
Dr. Andrew Robitschek
Dr. Kapuir

American Cancer Society
Heidi Williams
Becki Nunez

Wynette Smith
Mary Lipinski
Jacque Killibrew

Marilyn Schmidt*
Karen and Wes Weems

Robin and Don Johnson
Julie* and Greg Macedo
Roslyn Strohl*
Melody Lopez-Avant
Tim Ferrari
Krishanda Struble*
Heidi Struble-photographer
Laurie and Bill Struble

Mike Casey-pro surfer/assistant to writer
Larissa Franck-cover design
Jeanette Morris-editor
Karen Scott-web page design
Jim Hockin-watercolorist/cover design

BOOK ONE

COLLEGE DAYS

College days
Away from home
For the first time
All I want to do
Is have some fun
Tell dad I'll be OK
Don't worry, mom
Love, Amber
~This is a good day to live~

Chapter 1

<u>Say Goodbye</u>

Sunday, October 2, 1994

"On Saturday, we took our baby to her college in San Diego," I spoke bravely. "She's all settled into her dorm. It's going to be a wonderful experience for her." Across the wires, my mother couldn't see my splotchy, mascara stained cheeks. The tears made brown tracks running from my eyes. This was a not-so-unusual reaction for most parents sending their first-born child away from home for the first time. "She looked so excited and vulnerable when we left her," I added. That's when I cracked. I felt fresh tears spilling over the already red-rimmed eyes. This was by far the hardest and most painful thing I had ever done as a parent, aside from putting her on the school bus at age six.

Looking back, having Amber away was a huge adjustment. In the mornings when I would pass by her empty bedroom, I felt empty, too. I shed an avalanche of tears that first few weeks she was gone. Each day that passed my sadness came and went. I was disconsolate, but that had to be ok. Life happened so fast, one minute childhood, the next off to college to be an adult. I prayed every day for Amber and for the strength to let go of her with love. I missed her smile and her hugs so much. I remember thinking; I must be a good mother to feel so bad.

Our younger daughter, Bridgett, was excited to finally be the "only" child living at home with us. At fifteen, she would get our full attention at last. But, I'm sure she wasn't counting on her mother being so moody. I reminded her this too would pass, but I knew I was hanging by a thread.

Monday, October 10, 1994

Today, I take a deep breath. I had a pretty good day, but yesterday was an emotional one for me. Amber called and had an array of problems—seemingly insurmountable. I felt so good being her rescuer, then I got off the phone and blamed God for not cutting her any slack. I was replacing my sadness and built up anxieties with anger. Today, I made amends to God and with his help, I can go on and this too shall pass. I miss Amber so much and each time she calls, I feel more like my own mother to me. I am beginning to accept the fact that she is gone, and that is a positive step, but I go back to sadness in the next moment.

When she talks to me, I hear how tired she is and overwhelmed with her school work load, work study job at the football office, and juggling study time in between—of course time for fun is a concern for her as well. She has the world on her shoulders, but I keep reminding her to take pieces at a time. My heart goes out to her—new environment, new friends, new job, new teachers. It must really be a mountain for her. I wish I could help somehow. So, I baked her some cookies today and am preparing a care package for her. I want to help her feel at home somehow. I feel the tears coming again, and even though I've been doing OK so far today when I sit alone, in the quiet with no distractions, I realize underneath I'm still so sad.

I have fewer bad days now than the last time I wrote about my sadness over Amber leaving. As they say, time heals and life goes on, this too shall pass and all the other slogans that have been keeping me going for the last few weeks. She has been gone four weeks now—the longest time I've ever been separated from my child since her birth. She calls on a regular basis and last week was a little down over a biology test she had taken. She is placing a lot of pressure on herself to succeed. I reminded her that she has gone through a lot of changes in four weeks, and to expect that to affect her study habits.

I pray that she can keep up her pace of study and work—something she has never had to do before—and still be able to enjoy her new experiences of being on her own. Sometimes, I think she is too young and inexperienced to handle all of this—she just turned 18 barely two months ago. At this age, I was still at home with my family and friends surrounding me. I just keep praying that God watches over her, and that his will is something I can accept and live with.

Away

While you were sleeping
I gazed upon your face
The aura of Angels
hovered in grace
I watched while in slumber
the delicate hues
I sat down in wonder
what marvels I viewed
I reached out to touch you
then stopped in the air
the picture so perfect
of one that's so fair
So gently I lifted
myself from the bed
I smiled at the vision
there lying instead
I held to that memory
without my control
the picture of innocence
heart
mind
and
soul

Janine

October 12, 1994

Dear Mom,

Hi mommy! I felt bad tonight after talking to you guys about not writing, so I hurried and finished my homework so I'd have some extra time to write you all letters. I'm sorry that I haven't done it sooner.

I can't believe that I get to go home in about 10 more days. That's nothing. I know it will go by fast. I am so excited to be able to sleep in my own bed and be around my family who I've missed so much. I wish it could be for longer than a weekend, but I'll take what I can get. Besides being homesick every now and then, I really like my college. I think I made a good choice by coming here. I'm starting to make more girlfriends, too. I recently have become good friends with that girl Abby that I went out with for her birthday. She's super sweet! We have a lot of things in common and we both hang out with the same group of guys. Her roommate, Betty, is also really nice.

As far as a guy situation, there isn't one. Guys suck! Kurt claims he wants to visit me this coming Saturday, but I'm not getting my hopes up.

How's school for you? Is math going good? I hope better than my math. (end of subject, I know it's a bad one.)

Well, I gotta go to bed. I miss you tons and can't wait to spend time with you really soon. I love you,
Amberley
ps Give kitten a neck rub for me :)

Thursday, November 23, 1994

It's been a great Thanksgiving. I have a lot to be thankful for. Amber got home on Wednesday night about 7:45. She had experienced a lot of traffic coming from San Diego home. I was thinking about her and praying for her all day. She got home tired and happy. I can't get over how she is growing up. I would have never driven on the California freeways when I was her age.

She is still my sweet little girl, but to everyone else she is a young adult woman. She got a parking ticket (that makes two) and someone stole her tag on her license plate, so a ticket for that also. So, she's learning about life the hard way, just like we did. She stayed out with her friends until 3:30 am this morning. I slept OK, but Tom stayed awake most of the night and confronted her about it today. She defended herself pretty well, so he didn't get too far. Tom and I had a long talk about it. I told him he needs to detach with love, and telling her not to drink or stay up late or party too hard won't keep her from experimenting. She will have to learn the hard way—we can only show our disapproval, but she has to make her own decisions about what is right or wrong for her. He told her we wouldn't finance a big party. If she wants to be free to do that, she can come home. Well, she continued to defend herself—saying he was making a lot of untrue assumptions about her campus life. So, on and on, but we still love her. I love her so much and am already missing her smile before she ever leaves. I must remember she'll be home soon—six weeks at Christmas. I can't wait.

Amber's Story

Thursday, December 1, 1994

I was given this journal by my mom this weekend, which happened to be Thanksgiving weekend, upon my return home from college. My mom thought it would be good to record my thoughts and feelings throughout my first year in college. I happen to agree. Sometimes it's hard not being able to get out all that I keep bottled up inside. No one understands all that one goes through adjusting to a new life. College is tough...Both academically and emotionally. I don't feel like I'm an adult yet, but I know that I'm not a kid. So far, I've made some pretty bad judgment calls and can say I'm learning the hard way. Each time I feel like I'm letting someone down. Mostly my parents. This weekend I experienced the true seriousness of drinking under age. This is something that occurs quite often at college. I was naive to think I would always get away with it. To my surprise, I received a "minor in possession" for having alcohol in my car. Making yet another bad decision led to another let down in my parents eyes. It's not the actual ticket that gives me a sick feeling, but the fact that my dad and mom thought I was above that. I told the truth as far as whose it was (the liquor) and I believe this helped a little as far as demonstrating my responsibility, but as far as trust, once again it will have to be rebuilt.

Not only were my parents let down this weekend, but I, too, experienced a few disappointments. My friends seem so much more distant these days. I was warned that my relationships with them would change once I went away, but I never imagined that they would pull away as much as they have. It hurts to be walked on and ignored. I've decided to let go and accept them for who they are and what they've become, but it doesn't make it hurt any less. Sometimes I wish I could go back in time when life was so much simpler. I miss being able to have my parents and family there to take over when I couldn't handle it. Being able to cry on their shoulders when I had a bad day and when something good happened, being able to let them know first. I miss being a kid, I guess, is what it boiled down to. I hate having to deal with all of these stresses, problems and feelings all on my own.

One thing I've noticed about life away from home is the fact that my life is either up or down, there is never a happy medium. Today I was in a positive mood. It really wasn't due to any particular thing, but I woke up with the objective to make the most of my day. I've pretty much pushed the incident of this weekend out of my head and am trying not to worry about it for the time being. I had the opportunity to speak to Kurt this evening and we had an uplifting talk, which left a smile on my face. It's funny how something so small can make a difference.

Finals week is quickly approaching and once again I've found myself unprepared. Having to focus the majority of the week on little make-up assignments left me at Thursday in which I have to study for five tests. College is just one big stress in a series of roller coaster movements. I'm beginning to wonder if I'll be able to deal with it for the next 4-6 years of my life. At times I get really discouraged and feel as though it would be so much easier to quit school and just work, but then I'm reminded of how my future would look, very bare and trapping.

Sometimes I wonder if I suffer from a type of depression. Since I have been in San Diego, I find it harder and harder to find reasons to smile. I look at everything in a negative way and end up coming back to my room and crying.

I think the reason for this could have to do with being lonely. I look around and sometimes it seems like "everyone" has "someone" except me. I want so much to fall in love. When I start to think of this I can't handle my life anymore. I've made some mistakes in life that are going to reflect how some perceive me. This includes a big mistake made at this college with a guy named Mike. After my relationship with him, I don't think anyone will be interested in me for a long time. This is what my biggest fear and possibly the root of my anger. At times I begin to think things have blown over, then something is thrown before me to make me remember as well as others. He is the main reason for the prolonged situation because of his immaturities, but he will continue to affect my life for many months to come. What makes matters worse is he has ruined my chances with someone whom I care a lot for. This frustrates me because it is completely unfair.

So, added to my finals I have all of this shit to worry about, which leaves me as an unbearable individual to be around. I'm completely moody and on the verge of tears all times of the day. I think that it would probably help to see someone and talk about all of my inner feelings going on inside my head, but time is tight right now and therefore it's impossible. So the best I can do is write all of these feelings out on paper, which is what I'm doing. For the time being it's helping me to avoid being depressed so I guess it's working.

Saturday, December 17, 1994

Amber is home—yea! It's so nice having her smiling face around. She drove home without incident on Saturday. I am complete. All this makes me more grateful for my happy little family and that we are all together once again. Praise God!

We have been doing Christmas shopping, and so far I've been pretty successful for finding what I want. We are planning our trip to New Mexico and I'm getting excited to see everyone, especially my mom.

Sunday, December 18, 1994

I successfully completed the most stressful week of my life...finals week. I had a total of five finals being one a day for five days. To top things off, I got the flu the day before my first final and was sick for the week. I felt like giving up time and time again. I called my parents various times in tears because I didn't think I could make it, but I did. As far as my grades, I'll find out in a couple of weeks, which I'll have to deal with when the time comes. I think my biggest help during the week was the thought that soon enough I was going to be home for 6 weeks, with my parents and sister. This thought gave me the strength to continue on and not give up.

Now that I'm home I'm expecting another big adjustment. Rules and having to let my parents know where I'm going and when I'll be home. This will be tough. I'm so used to controlling my own life that having parents, in this aspect, will be tough. Other than this, I'm extremely excited to be home for a while and to not have to worry about school.

Bridgett

Softly, as she sleeps
I peek in and get a glimpse of
this child
of mine
Her dimpled eyes
and sun kissed nose
I catch her lying
in sweet repose
It's my treat
to see her innocence
Vulnerable, at last
no barriers there
Only me and her
against a crooked world
I watch as she sleeps
and marvel
She is mine

Mother's Day 1996
Janine

Bridgett's Journal
Friday, December 30, 1994

I know I haven't written in a while, I guess I just never thought about it. I am a sophomore in high school now and I think I finally realized that I am growing up. I promise myself right now that for the New Year I am going to try and write in this book as much as possible. I think it will help me clear my head.

Well, today we just got back from New Mexico. I had a pretty good time. I would have liked to stay longer. My grandfather was put in the hospital and it was a little scary. It just made me realize when it's your time, it's your time. No, it wasn't my grandpa's time. I think God knows that he is still very much needed by my grandmother. I also think that it was a wake-up call to my Grandma Verna reminding her how much she loves and needs him.

Life is still just a mystery to me. I just have my theories of what or how I think it is. (That is, the purpose of life.)

The other day, Sunday, at church, Father Ron told a story that made me really think. It was about how God talks to you in many ways. He won't just pop into your life and say, "I'm here." He gives you signs and signals. You, yourself have to be aware, waiting for these signs. I think this is one of the few times I actually listened at church. I think I'm beginning to realize the significance of religion. I still don't always want to go to church, but I just have so many questions about Jesus, God and everything. I'm interested. Anyway, I will write more later.   BC

Monday, January 2, 1995

Our whirlwind trip is over and now it's time to start a new year. The plane arrangements were a bad experience and one I wouldn't like to repeat. The visit to Albuquerque was successful and fulfilling, however, like having a baby, I wouldn't want to do it every day! We got there on the 26th and left on the 30th. For the amount of time we spent there, it was very expensive and we really only had three days to visit anyone. We were all exhausted after the trip.

One of the last nights we were there, Mom had a Christmas party for the entire family...all 31 of us. The atmosphere was jovial and loud and everyone was catching up on each other's lives. Our little family was the star attraction because we are the only ones that live out of state. It was a lot of fun, and just plain a lot of everything.

During the party, Amber noticed a lump near her collarbone. Mom took a look at it and became slightly alarmed. She made me vow that I would take her to the doctor as soon as possible when we got home. The lump is uncomfortable for Amber, but not painful. So, we shall see about that soon.

With the exception of poor travel arrangements on my part, the trip was great. I am renewed for another year, but another trip during the holidays is out for me! I look forward to a new semester at Allan Hancock College and hope I'll get accepted to Cal Poly. Tom is still not working, so seeking work out of town seems to be the next step for him.

Friday, January 6, 1995

Amber saw the doctor today at 1:30. She has never seen this woman before, and was a little anxious, but still wanting to find out what this lump is all about. The doctor thinks it is a swollen thyroid nodule. She will have blood work done on Friday, results by Tuesday. I pray it is not serious.

Wednesday, January 11, 1995

Today, our family went to Amber's ultra sound appointment at the hospital. It took about an hour. The doctor will have results by tomorrow. Seeing the pictures of that lump on the screen makes it seem real—now we wait to see the diagnosis. Again I pray it's nothing serious. It is very tense around here because of this test and our uncertainty.

The clouds are following us. Amber's court appearance is tomorrow at 1:00 pm for the Minor in Possession she received for having an open container of alcohol in the parking lot of the Grad nightclub. Even though I see this as simply "growing pains," getting caught has created more anxiety. God grant me serenity… I am anxious to start school—I wish I started after Amber, though. I want to spend as much time with her as possible. Tom is projecting her departure and is sorrowful already. I am going to try and stay in today so I can enjoy her as much as I can for the time we have left together.

Saturday, January 13, 1995

Yesterday Amber had her wisdom teeth pulled and it was quite an ordeal for all of us. I went in to be with her as the drug put her to sleep. The last words on her lips were, "I love you, Mommy." She was my little girl again and in her helpless state she reverted back before my very eyes to the sweet young child I have raised. These things I hold near to my heart. Amber is truly my special one. She gives me great joy and great sorrow. I feel the sorrow as I write today. I'm thinking of how it will be when she again goes back to school. Even though she has matured in many ways, she still has a quality of softness and vulnerability that makes me feel close to her.

She has such thoughtful ways. I am beside myself with anxiety over the growth on her neck. The doc has now referred her to an ear, nose, and throat specialist. She thinks it's her lymph nodes. There are two of them next to the thyroid. I am mad because this process takes so long. I am filled with "what ifs." The big one is cancer. God help me to visualize this as only benign cysts that can be removed simply and finally. I fear, so I must renew my faith. I pray and let it go, and then I take it back. I must continue to pray. So far, the two previous crises have had mild finales. Her court appearance was a two-hour wait and then a $135 fine of a city ordinance infraction. That was a relief to her, no license revoked, as she had feared. Secondly, she is recovering nicely from the tooth surgery—not much swelling, no profuse bleeding, mostly pain and discomfort. Tom and I were by her side every moment. Even Bridgett stayed home last night to be with her sister. She is showing some signs of jealousy. I must admit, we are paying a lot of attention to Amber at this time, but rightly so.

Thursday, January 19, 1995

This has been the week from hell. I had a major confrontation with the staff at Dr. Whippet's office about Amber's HMO insurance referral and started my period this morning, just in time for my first day back to school!! I am not a happy camper. Looming over my head now is Amber's appointment with the ear, nose and throat specialist about the lumps in her neck. She goes in today. Tom will go with her since I have school until 3:00. I pray that these things are just cysts that can be reduced with medications. The doctor said it was her lymph nodes, whatever that means.

Amber mentioned to me yesterday that she is re-thinking about attending the University of San Diego for the rest of her college time. Two of her friends at Chico State are thinking about attending a junior college for a while. This has her thinking, too. I'm not getting my hopes up, but the seed is planted. She will still go back for this semester, but who knows after that. I am missing her smile already. She has become dependent on us through her illnesses and I think she wants to stay home. I don't blame her. It's so far away to San Diego.

I hope I have good news when next I write.

Sunday, January 22, 1995

Today, Tom goes to San Francisco to work on a refinery. He will have three days off each weekend, so at least he'll be home one more day than expected. I am ambivalent about his leaving. It has always been difficult to be the single parent when he's gone. Right now I need him here. He's been home for a while now, but when he doesn't work, he doesn't get paid. It is necessary for him to go and I can accept that. I cannot accept the uncertainty I still feel about all of these test results for Amber.

The mononucleosis test was negative, and now we must have a needle aspiration procedure done at the hospital next week. It will be a biopsy. I fear for her and I honestly don't feel very optimistic about her condition anymore. This week will give us the long awaited information. She is so tired of these tests, and I don't blame her. She's been poked and stabbed enough. So, I will be with her through all the process. Tom will be here in spirit. He feels bad that he can't be here with her. That's why there are two parents. I will be right there with Amber, no matter what. She will need my care and support to get through this ordeal. I will call on the support of my higher power.

Monday, January 23, 1995

A mother's worst fear is that her child will have an illness that is serious. My worst fear has come true. Amber has been diagnosed with cancer—there, I've said it. It is a scary bogeyman that creeps around in darkness and claims its victim, innocent and undeserving of such a fate. I have cried many times since Dr. Steward broke the news to Amber and me in his small office. In all his wisdom, he found the words to tell a mother and daughter the most dreaded news.

Amber was so helpless looking as she asked him, "Is this bad?" Her frightened look, her quivering voice; my worst nightmare had come true. As we made our way into the parking lot, the rain began to fall, from the skies, from our eyes. My baby, sweet baby, what's to become of you? Her words to me, pleading and filled with fear were, "I don't want to die!" God, be merciful; she is so young and has so much to do and feel and love and experience. I tried to find the words to comfort her, but all I could do was bravely assure her that she was not going to die. But first, I had to believe it myself and I just wasn't sure anymore what to pray for.

In the darkness of the wet and fear filled night, we held onto each other in the front seat of the car. Eventually I had to drive, but I don't remember much about driving. I held her hand until we got home. I had to keep my faith that she would be OK and recover.

I found myself remembering a week ago how I would miss Amber so terribly when she went back to college. And now I was wishing she were normal and getting ready to go back and enjoy her college life and classes and young friends and experience.

I must call my mom...I want to hear her voice. I need mothering. I need my husband who is working out of town right now. I had to break the bad news to him yesterday over the phone. He was devastated. At first he was rushing home, but I talked him out of driving while he was so upset.

This is so hard to accept. I still can't believe this is happening. These things happen in the movies, not for real. My God, have mercy. Jay, who is the youth minister of our church and a personal friend of both my girls, called tonight to share his concern. I don't know how he found out about Amber's diagnosis, but he offered to talk to Fr. Ron tomorrow on her behalf. I want to have him give Amber a special blessing and say a mass for her. This pain shall pass...I have to keep the faith.

I am so tired. Today I called my extended family to tell them the dreaded results of the tests done on Amber. It was so emotional. I am mentally exhausted. So many questions I could not answer. I requested that each person write down 21 personal positive affirmations on Amber's behalf. It was the only constructive thing I could think of that they could do to feel helpful.

Dr. Steward telephoned today. The surgery to remove the two lymph nodes will be on Friday morning. He talked to Amber briefly and answered all our collective questions. I feel better, yet drained from all the crying and explaining I had to do for hours this morning. I feel like crawling into bed and staying there with the covers pulled over my head. Each day the pieces of the puzzle come together. By Monday, we should know the facts of his preliminary diagnosis of Hodgkin's disease. I'll be glad when we know more.

BOOK TWO

HOSPITAL DAYS

Hospital days
Away from home
For the second time
All I want to do
Is live
Tell dad I'll be OK
Don't worry, mom
Love, Amber
~This is a good day to live~

Chapter One

<u>New Doctor</u>

Friday, January 27, 1995

    We are waiting in the cafeteria of the hospital. The tables are big, the seats are cold, and there is a draft over my right shoulder. Is it the coffee I've had this morning, or am I finally just in some form of acceptance that makes me feel content? I am waiting for Amber to come out of her biopsy surgery. I can't believe it has come to this, and then I am brought to reality and I know where I am and why.

    We have been up since 4:30 am, so I'm a little scattered in my thoughts, but I know what I feel. Hopeful. Amber was very positive as she was wheeled into the surgery room at 7:00am. Dr. Steward will remove the lumps and the tests will show what she has. My prayer is that he has the news I want to hear—that he got all of the yucky stuff out and it hasn't spread. I have trust and confidence that this will be true. I hate the wait and it's been one hour since she went in. Bridgett is holding up all right, but Tom is still in the "why" stage. His tears are coming and that's good. I have been through that and moving onto the next stage—Amber's recovery from surgery, and final diagnosis and treatment plan.

    She was smiling as she was wheeled into surgery. She took my childhood rosary in with her, taped to her arm. I told her to feel my hand in hers. I asked her what she wanted to take in with her. She said, " Your hand would be nice." She is so brave.

It is 9:00 am and the doctor came to consult with us. He removed three lymph nodes, but saw no other bad stuff while he was in there. They haven't read the chest x-ray yet, so there's no guarantee it's not in the chest nodes. The rest of the day was dedicated to helping Amber feel as comfortable as possible. Tom, Bridgett and I tried to do that for her. She has such courage and even gave us her famous smile. She has been through so much in the last few weeks. It breaks my heart to watch her struggle to sit up, to turn her head, to do anything that involves head movement. She's on pain meds, but she is still itching so much, a symptom of the disease, and it keeps her awake at night. My sweet baby—her life for a while will consist of doctors, tests, treatments, poking and prodding. I will be with her, of course, but her body must feel the pain, her brain must know the anxiety of waiting to hear about one more test. How much more are we in for? Dr. Steward is non-committal; it's out of his hands now and into Dr. Dan's, the oncologist. This is the big "kahuna" in the mysterious world of cancer whom we will finally see tomorrow. I am fearful today of what he will say to us. I am sharing my fear on paper—I can't let it show today. I know each of us will be holding our own fears of what will be. I will try not to think of it now.

We have lots of prayers coming our way from back home. I've made my last phone call to my old high school buddy, Donna, this morning. She was shaken, having heard the news from our mutual friend, Louise, first hand. They are both more than just friends to turn to, and I need their power through prayer.

Friday, February 2, 1995

Well, Monday was quite a day for us. We picked up x-rays and history from doctors Whippet and Steward to hand carry them to the new doctor's office. That was the business part of it. The emotional part of it was left out for the time being. I managed to be a good listener as Dr. Dan introduced himself to us. With the wisdom and forthrightness of a man twice his age, he proceeded to inform us of Amber's illness. He painted a positive picture, however, I saw it in drab and lifeless colors. We sat there as a family unit, hearing the details of Hodgkin's disease plotted out like an itinerary of someone's vacation plans. He was so positive that we were all lulled into acceptance, and before we knew it, he had us believing it was just a normal happening instead of a scary nightmare.

He had a serious, yet positive and even a little reckless manner about him. His experience with this sort of thing certainly showed through. Tears for me would not come until much later. Too many things to ask about, too much to mentally digest. Then, came the latest array of tortures…they call them tests; the bone marrow biopsy procedure. Resembling something the Japanese may have done to prisoners in WWII to squeeze information out of them; I held my baby's hand as he drilled holes in her back to remove bone marrow for testing the progression of the cancer. This had to be the worst part of the staging process. If the cancer cells are there, it will be very serious. We now have to wait three days for results. The waiting is so hard. Each test means one step closer to ending the staging process and the beginning of treatments to get rid of the evil cells growing in my child's body.

Thursday, February 7, 1995

Because of the possibility of there being lymph nodes affected in Amber's lungs, she has been scheduled for a C.A.T scan today. So here we sit, in the reception room of radiology, waiting for Amber to be called for her turn to be pushed through the giant tunnel that will perform this type of x-ray procedure. This should be painless, with the exception of an I.V. that has to be inserted. A doctor will then put dye into her vein, which will help outline the rest of her organs so they can pinpoint the lymph nodes.

This morning Amber is doing OK, but had a sleepless night due to the combination of anxiety and the barium she had to drink that made her gut hurt. She is more concerned about the results than the actual procedure. This staging process is so grueling, and the waiting is unbearable. This test will allow them to look and see if the disease has spread to her other lymph nodes in the chest, abdomen, or pelvic area. Once the procedure is over, we will go home to rest and then back to see Dr. Dan in his office to get the results of this and the bone marrow biopsy he performed on Monday.

While Amber is getting the C.A.T. scan done I am in the dressing room listening. She is alone in there—I hate that. I am as close to her as I can be. It must be scary for her even though the technician is very perky and nice. Her name is Lynn, and she will call me when the IV is to be put in, so I can be with her to hold her hand. The test will take 40 minutes. It's 11:20 now. We have been waiting since 9:15. I'm glad I asked my friend, Karen, to pick up Bridgett today from school. I would like to take Amber to lunch after this scan is over and go shopping for a pretty blouse or something. She has been through so much; it's the least I can do to cheer her up. I love her very much. I wish it were me instead of her having to go through this. She is so innocent and has really begun to cling to me. I stayed with her last night when she had trouble sleeping—it's such a little thing to do for her, I wish I could do much more. Take it all away at least. Right now I can hear her talking to the technician. She is laughing and it sounds good to my ears.

It is so strange how our lives outside all of this are still going on. Amber is enrolled in twelve units at Allan Hancock, one of the local community colleges. She has met with a nice counselor, Mr. English, who is making sure the classes she takes will articulate at USD when she goes back to school there. Higher education is of major importance to Amber. She is taking a ballet class there with me. We are becoming more than just mother and daughter. Now we are fellow students and friends.

Unfortunately, that is not the case at this time with Bridgett. We had a fight yesterday when I picked her up from school. She was in a fair mood, but it didn't last. I had dropped her at school for some cheerleading practice, and Amber and I went to the beach. It was so beautiful. The sun was shining, the sky clear. We walked in the water and just enjoyed being with each other. She had been stressing about possibly losing her hair if she had to have chemotherapy. I thought we needed to get out and feel good about something. It worked for a while to get her mind off of the grim reality.

Once picked up, Bridgett and I instantly fought—she was fifteen minutes late and I was hot and mad. One thing led to the next; at home there was shouting—she is feeling left out—she has a life—we really had to talk about this because her anger is the way she is coping with the way things are right now. I can intellectualize this, but emotionally I just get angry back. She is needy, but so am I. I think we can be helpers to each other now that we got that straight. We need each other. It is crucial we are on the same side. I love her.

Friday, February 3, 1995

The news from Dr. Dan wasn't good. Amber has a spot on her lung. More surgery is needed for a biopsy, and chemo is a sure thing now for treatment. Negative for cancer in the bone marrow, so at least that's positive news. We are all taking this pretty hard. I had my hopes that it was just in the neck and radiation would be the form of treatment, but now the prognosis isn't very good. More lengthy treatment will be necessary, and the dreaded chemo. The medical terms are used in a nonchalant manner in conversation now.

Amber's life is taking a real turn. She was devastated mainly by the fear of hair loss as a probable side effect of the chemotherapy treatment. She cried openly with Dr. Dan and he tried to show the positive side to all of this. "That spot on your lung could have been overlooked if the x-ray had been done too soon; now we can deal with it," he reminded her. Cancer is so evil it could be anywhere. That's the reason to poison her system to get rid of it all. Unfortunately, there is such a down side. I am scared for her. I must really be careful now to be strong and keep her positive. I just can't call all those people back home. I'm so weary of telling the details, answering all the questions; I can't handle that right now. I think I will just call my mom—I can't talk to anyone else about all of this.

Saturday, February 4, 1995

I have just read the sheet explaining Hodgkin's disease for the 100th time. As more questions arise about Amber's stage of the disease, I begin to want answers, so I read. Now her dad is angry because he would rather not know, and I can see his point of view; but it is not mine.

The needle aspiration will be done on Monday at 7:45 to establish what type of cancer the "spot" on her lung is. Instead of surgery, they will try and hit it with a needle to get it tested. For now, I can't worry about it. It is a weekend that I must try to be as normal as possible for all of us involved. I must try to not think of the worst and stay in today. Amber needs that from me.

Sunday, February 5, 1995

This is the night before Amber's next test. I went to church tonight with Bridgett, and Tom stayed home and cooked supper. Amber went out with Kurt. She is trying to be "normal" and I don't blame her. This test will be uncomfortable, but it should tell us more about her condition and stage of the disease. Tom is taking off work and going with us. It was his decision and his boss is supportive. Everyone is being very tolerant and mostly understanding. Some people are just pushy, like Abby's mom who wanted to know if we "explored all the possibilities" for the best care of Amber. What nerve! As though we wouldn't think to do the best for our daughter. I just don't understand this side of people. I don't even know this woman.

We prayed together tonight on the floor of our bedroom—Bridgett, Tom and I. It felt good to hold hands and feel God in our circle. Tonight I feel hopeful.

Chapter Two

<u>Staging process begins</u>

Monday, February 6, 1995

Here we sit, at French Hospital, waiting for Amber to be called in for the needle aspiration prep. I hate waiting, but it has to be done. She is worried and irritated this morning. Tom is with us today. Maybe she feels she can have her true feelings and she doesn't have to keep my spirits up since her dad is here with me. Anyway, I must keep positive thoughts and conversation going to help keep her mind off the anxiety of waiting—and to help me, too!

I was with Amber right up until the time the radiologist, Dr. Muller, put the needle in to remove the mysterious fluid from the tiny spot on her lung. It is remarkable how these things can be done. They placed a grid on Amber's chest made of metal wires, then the C.A.T. scan took the picture and while she was in the machine, he put the needle in the spot, one he found that was "much bigger," he said. Does this mean she has more than one affected node inside her lung?

About three inches into her body, he pulled out the cells through a tiny needle. This is truly awesome. He allowed me to be with her right up until he did the procedure. She looked so small and vulnerable inside that big machine. I have many pictures in my mind of her tests that I wish would go away—but this one is classically unforgettable. The giant tunnel they slipped her into dwarfed her size even more. There was my little girl being poked and prodded again. These doctors and nurses were very comforting—the doctor would pat my back as he would go by and the nurse, Lynne, was the one who held Amber's hand in my place when the needle went in. It seemed a short while before the doc came to the waiting area where I busied myself with my crochet on Amber's afghan. He was optimistic that he got a good sample. Tom questioned him about some stuff and I was getting impatient—I just wanted to be back with Amber. Shut up already.

When I went back in to see her, she was covered up with a green cotton towel up to her chin—a drop of blood on her chest was all that was left as a reminder of the delicate procedure. My heart was joyful to see her smile—a weak one, but a smile. We went back to x-ray, got one of her chest to see if her lung had collapsed, (thank heavens no), but the next three hours were spent in a tiny room in the ambulatory section of the hospital used for outpatients. It was a long, grueling day. Amber had an I.V. poked on top of her right wrist and it hurt her the whole time, but she made it through. Then, Dr. Dan came in to tell us the results of the biopsy. The lung is involved with Hodgkin's. I'm not sure what that means, but I am suspicious it isn't the news we wanted. At least there will be no more tests for staging purposes, and no more surgery. We have decided to seek out a second opinion and go from there.

Tuesday, February 7, 1995

This is quite a path we are going down. Dr. Dan is a very thorough, nice man-nered doctor, and I don't doubt him; it's just recommended to get a second opinion before any treatment begins. In a way I want to get started on treatment because I hate the thought of those bugs being inside Amber. I also know once it begins, there will be side effects we'll have to deal with that won't be pleasant. Hair loss, nausea, and vomit-ing are all possible adverse reactions, but not in all cases. Amber is constantly worried about her hair, hoping she will be the exception. She got pretty frustrated today. I think she needs to hit something and just get mad. I haven't seen her get mad yet. She cries a lot, maybe that's all she needs. I know I take out my anger on paper as I did with my poison pen letter about the referral fiasco with her primary care doctor's office. What a bunch of jerks, making us wait for a week for a referral. HMO's suck. I also write in this journal to clear my head. It helps a lot.

Next week we will probably be going to Pasadena to the City of Hope, a major medical center where they treat cancer patients. This is the next phase, then the treat-ment procedure. We need strength for what's to come. I think I need some extra prayers right now.

It has been over a month since this whole nightmare began. On January 6, Amber and I sat in the office of Dr. Whippet waiting her turn to be seen. It was an average day by most standards, but there was a feeling of apprehension as we waited patiently and as I stayed in the reception area while Amber saw the doc alone. I stayed behind, thinking I needed to let her be the adult she wanted to be and that she may have personal questions and needed her privacy. In retrospect, I see that was a mistake of gigantic proportions. When she came out with orders to get some blood work done, my heart sank. How could I have known this was only the beginning of needle poking, x-rays, and medical tortures beyond my belief? That our naive, yet "wanting to be grown up" little girl had cancer as we sat there waiting for her blood to be drawn? I am remembering the fear in her eyes and apprehension of the first needle, and the quick squeeze of her hand around mine as the dirty deed was being done. Then, the worst part of all that we never get accustomed to: waiting...

We are certainly on a journey. Next stop, City of Hope, probably on Monday. The referral has been approved—no longer do these papers sit on someone's desk forgotten—they are now marked "urgent" as they should have been from the very beginning. And now, we wait...and when we get there, we will wait...and I will get Amber's afghan finished, for every square now has new meaning—thoughts of love and inspiration fill my head as my fingers busy themselves and give my eyes something to stare at. My admiration for Amber is great. She holds on to a peaceful, positive attitude, wise beyond her years. Thoughts and actions bathed in tears, buckets of them by now. She is afraid of losing her hair. I wish I could guarantee that won't happen, but I can't. If it does, she will bear it with the strength it took to get this far and her will to be cured of this evil thing. This is truly a lesson in humility for all of us. That we are so smug in thinking we have our lives so neatly planned out.

Interlude

"Thank heaven for little girls." Maurice Chevalier sang for the millionth time. I had been creating a ballet for our ballerina threesome, Amber, Bridgett and mommy. The recital was three weeks away and the choreography was finally finished. Now came the hard part, to perform it and to "sell" it to the audience. How do you get to Carnegie Hall? Practice, practice, practice.

Amber was eight and Bridgett five, but the three years of experience Amber had over her sissy didn't affect Bridgett at all. She was all the more diligent to learn the steps she'd never done before.

"*Pas-de-booo-ree*," I emphasized the "boo" and placed my feet in fifth position just so. "We all have to be here on count three."

Oh, those little feet attached to those cute legs, topped off with those tiny *derrière's*. Bridgett wiggled hers to get the tight position required of all famous ballerinas. Fonteyne had nothing on my girls.

"But, Mom, you said on count four we would be here," countered my Amber as she demonstrated.

"Yes, originally it was like that," I agreed, "but now I want the *relevé* to be on count three instead. That will give us the four full counts of the measure to finish the phrase." I had to show her I knew a little more than she did about choreography, although, I had to admit proudly that she was beginning to show a flair for creating *enchainment*.

There was still a lot of work to be done to polish the number, but the countless hours spent at the dance studio only bonded us together and made our relationship as mother and daughters closer than an average family. We could always count on dad to be in the audience clapping and praying for a good performance.

Whenever we performed this number, all the mothers in the audience would have tears in their eyes. I must admit it gave me great pride to dance with my two darling daughters. As a mother it was the epitome of accomplishment. Not only were my girls talented, they wanted to dance with me. That made my heart burst with happiness. It was the highest honor I ever received aside from giving them life.

Chapter Three

Second opinion

Monday, February 13,1995

    We are at the City of Hope Hospital in Duarte, CA. After a three-hour drive from home, our tight little family peel themselves out of the car one by one and step into a huge parking lot to gaze at the center where hope is supposed to live.

    I'm feeling more anxiety than hope right now as we embark on yet another path toward this "less traveled road." Bridgett and Amber walk ahead as a duo joined by their hands. Tom and I follow. For a moment I flash back on family trips to Sea World or miniature golf. A thousand more pleasant memories of days spent on excursions together. Then, the harsh reality of where we are and why. This is a cancer treatment hospital, and it looms before us like Jonah's whale with its mouth open, ready to swallow us all in one fatal gulp.

    We enter through the front doors, and are immediately thrown into a lion's den of white lab coats and patients of every possible age in every possible mode of transportation; wheel chairs, walkers, gurneys. People with no hair shuffling by, pulling their IV poles, and wheeling them around like their dog on a leash, oblivious to these outsiders that we are. We stare into the sea of faces mingling in the huge arena known as the waiting area.

I gather my strength and tell my family to find a seat as I forge on to the semi-circle counter that is referred to as "check in." Refusing to let my small stature and wide eyes divulge any weakness, I bravely announce our arrival.

"My daughter, Amber Carter is here to have a consult." I push the words out.

"Who's her doctor?" the clerk asks crisply.

"Dr. Spyberg. We are here for a second opinion. Here is her insurance referral."

"Have a seat. You are number 81."

Dismissed.

I find my welcomed nest of three waiting, huddled together against the storm of other patients and caregivers lined along the walls, seated and waiting for their number to come up. Meanwhile, we gaze out into the multitude of bodies and do some people watching to pass the time. This is quite a scene. TV's perched high in the corners of the holding room, and a large board with numbers, some lit up. Apparently, that's when we'll know it's our turn. This is sort of like bingo, only the winner gets her blood drawn. We share our attention between people watching, TV watching, and number watching.

Amber sees her number light up. The next step is to get her blood drawn for tests and her vital signs checked. We walk against the waves of people, bonded together like the last episode of the Mary Tyler Moore Show when they hug en masse and scoot as a group to answer the telephone.

We are directed to a long corridor with signs above different rooms, and lines of people in front of each one. When it is Amber's turn to have her blood drawn, I go with her into the cubical. I hold her hand while lab techs poke and suck her blood into a vial. I tell her to squeeze my hand and put her pain into it, wishing she really could. Our visit to Dr. Spyberg is a brief and somber meeting. He casually mentions the fact that once chemotherapy has begun, she will likely become infertile. That is like dropping a bomb on a hospital full of children with my child inside. I have to file that bit of information into the dark recesses of my brain until I can really think about its repercussions.

We are hearing the same litany Dr. Dan has already told us about Hodgkin's disease. Because there is involvement in a major organ, the lung, she is categorized as Stage IV. No doubt more details will be revealed in the days to come, but right now she is being prepped for another excruciating bone marrow biopsy. Why they have to do another one of those is beyond me. We could have hand carried the bone marrow collected by Dr. Dan and that should have been enough. Too late to think of this, and again she suffers as we all become witnesses to another painful procedure. Again my hand becomes a vehicle for a minute piece of her pain.

The City of Hope panel of 14 physicians will discuss Amber's case and give their professional opinion. If the general consensus is matched to Dr. Dan's diagnosis, she will begin chemotherapy immediately. We should have these results by Wednesday.

We were all quite ready to head on home to our little town by the sea. As we approached that welcomed sight, it began to rain. Like the clouds, we felt the release of the tension of the long and arduous day.

Saturday, February 18, 1995

Today my heart is heavy. Amber has been down since our trip, feeling blue, and seems to have little energy. Her guy friend, Kurt, hasn't called and her friends are being flaky. Funny how that alone can put her into a depression. If I had cancer, I would certainly be that way, too. But, it seems like for her, it is the rejection of friends that puts her over the edge. Tom and I took her to the beach; it was a beautiful sunny day. That helped for a while, but when we got home she positioned herself on the couch and stayed there the rest of the day. Actually, I did get her out again to do some shopping. I think I may be having trouble with acceptance myself. I don't like the way God is putting her through this. I wish she could be like other kids her age, worrying about school tests instead of medical ones. She talks about Sandra going with her friends to Lake Havasu for spring break. She can't do those things with what is on her agenda: doctor's visits, chemotherapy, ill effects from treatment—this will be our world—and it sucks. I need to pray more so I won't feel this way.

Chapter Four

<u>Amber speaks out</u>

Sunday, February 12, 1995

A lot has changed in my life since the last time I wrote down my thoughts. Basically my life has been turned upside-down. Upon my return home from college for Christmas, I discovered a lump on my neck and after which I was supposed to return to school, I have had 28 needles poked in virtually every part of my body. Starting with my neck, which ended in surgery to remove the cancerous lymph nodes. This was when I found out for sure it was Hodgkin's. From then I had to go to a cancer doctor and begin the "staging" process, beginning with a bone marrow sampler, which was very painful, then C.A.T. scans, then a needle biopsy of my lung. Now I've been told I am at the 4th stage and have probably had this for about 6-8 months.

It has been a tough adjustment to cope with the fact that I have cancer. My first questions were "Why me?" and "Am I going to die?" From what Dr. Dan says, I'm not going to die, but he can't answer the first question, only God can.

Through my discovery of the disease, I have begun to realize who really are my true friends and they all happen to be away from me. This leaves me feeling alone a lot of the time. I sit and think a lot and though I know negative energy is bad for me, I have a hard time being my happy self again. I miss the old life I used to lead and basically <u>having</u> a life. All I really have to look forward to is 8 months down the road before I will be able to be normal again.

Chemotherapy is what is scaring me the most. The side effects are going to be awful, but hair loss is a small price to pay for my life.

I thank God for my family and my best friend, Sandra. I don't know what I would do without them.

Monday, February 13, 1995

It's the day before Valentine's Day and again I am beginning to feel more and more alone. The one friend I felt I could depend on is also distancing himself from me.

Not only do I have a disease, but also I'm beginning to feel like one. Every friend I have left, who isn't away at college, has dwindled out of my life. I was starting to believe that Kurt was a gift from God to help me through this rough time. Now, all he seems to be concerned with is not letting me get the wrong idea and tie him down. All I need is a close friend to be there for me! I feel as though the world is a bubble and I'm on the outside looking in. It's awful to feel alone and it's the worst thing for my health, but I feel like I'm on a downhill slope...My only hope is someone who is willing to always be there for me and give me a hand. I can't handle all of these feelings and emotions alone any longer.

I'm hoping that my therapist can find a girl or boy my age that is going through the same thing and knows how I'm feeling. Once this is accomplished, I think I will begin to feel less abnormal. I miss being like everyone else!

Tuesday, February 14, 1995

Well, today was Valentine's Day and unexpectedly, I received a box of chocolates from Kurt. Although I would have rather seen him and spent quality time with him, it was a thoughtful gift that let me know we still have a good friendship. Pretty much, today was a good day. I got out and got exercise at a ballet class and began redoing my bedroom. I find that when I'm busy I don't dwell on my hardships as much. It, in turn, helps my overall attitude of life for that day. It's funny how touch and go it can sometimes be, but I'm living day by day and today was good.

Wednesday, February 15, 1995

Yesterday was a pretty good day. Amber was able to take an entire ballet class. She also got a valentine from Kurt and that sent her to bed smiling. It didn't happen so easily. There were some tears when she thought he hadn't remembered her, but after a little talk with me, I convinced her that it is a joy to give as well as receive. She went to Kurt's house and took him a valentine and lo and behold, he was just coming over to see her with one! She has such expectations and she gives up quickly. Not so with the disease—she is still fairly optimistic about that, even marginally accepting possible hair loss.

I shared at my support meeting last night that I know I am in for a few hard weeks to come. I will call Dr. Spyberg today for the consensus of opinion at City of Hope. Then, we will meet with Dr. Dan to start chemo. I'm anxious about that. I can only imagine how it will be. So, I must pray, put one foot in front of the other, and hang on tight for the next bumpy ride. I've dropped several hints to my mom for her to come be with us. I think I could use her help right now.

Friday, February 17, 1995

Amber and I just came from Sierra Vista hospital for a gallium scan, the latest test to determine the stage of Hodgkin's disease. She was loaded up with radioactive isotopes yesterday by injection, and now this will collect in the areas of Hodgkin's disease in her system. Spyberg and his associates at the City of Hope felt the test should be done and Dr. Dan agreed. So, now she's radioactive! They will check by scanning her on a special machine on Saturday and Sunday, to see where the isotopes collected. Supposedly that is where the cancer would be.

Wait more, worry more. I'm dreaming about this stuff. I wake up with it, live it, and go to bed with it. Writing helps to sort out my feelings. Sometimes I look at her and I just see Amber—not any different, but those moments are brief. I am thankful that there is no outward appearance, but even with that likelihood, I will always think of her as a beautiful, loving child. She has to put her life on hold for a while. Her best friend, Sandra, is coming to stay with us this weekend and I'm so glad for that.

With the help of her friend, Amber will get through this difficult period. My high school buddy, Donna, lives close to USD and is coming this weekend to bring Amber's stuff from her college dormitory. I can't thank her enough for stepping up to our cause. My life seems so out of whack—I'm trying to maintain school, but it's getting out of control. I have no regimen, study time, etc. I missed class on Thursday to go with Amber for the injection to begin the gallium scans. Her needs come first and school is an afterthought. I didn't apply to Cal Poly for the spring as I need to be flexible with my time. My priorities have changed.

I ran the rehearsal for Bridgett's dance company at the high school last night. It was good to be needed by someone outside my small world. It was fun to watch them and give them pointers; I felt very welcomed. I will go today at school and help out again—this way I can show some interest and support in what Bridgett is doing. She needs that from me now. Tom and I see our family therapist on Sunday and that will be good for us. Maybe we can go to Montana De Oro afterwards and sit by the ocean's surf. Some quality R and R is much needed.

Tuesday, February 21, 1995

There seems to be a lack of time for all I need to do. I'm feeling a little over-whelmed because of paperwork from USD (I'm trying to get an extension on Amber's leave of absence from classes) scholarship applications, letters from my complaint to Dr. Whippet's office about the referral nightmare, Amber's loan extension forms, income taxes, bills to be paid. I'm just on overload right now. I shouldn't complain, these are such trivial things compared to Amber's health. The gallium scan didn't give the infor-mation needed about the lung spots. Now, she has to have another needle stuck in her lung and Dr. Muller will try to hit the spot that's two centimeters in size. Here we go again. These tests are wearing me down. I can't plan on anything, or get any kind of routine going. We never know what test will be next. My prayer is that he gets a good sample and Dr. Dan can find out what he needs to know from it without having to request surgery to remove the spot from her lung. "Wait" is the name of this game. What about me? I'm tired of the whole mess, but I must keep my chin up for Amber's sake.

Meanwhile, we went wig shopping yesterday. Amber looks so cute with short hair. She was in a good mood and I had to hold my mother's tears back. She is daunt-less. I hope I can be this brave for the next steps to come. I need hope; I need to know that the white light at the end of the tunnel is there for her and me.

Chapter Five

<u>More tests for staging</u>

Friday, February 24, 1995

    Opting for a second opinion was my choice, and now I'm realizing how much more precise they have to be. I had to get a gallium scan, which concluded to be just as they originally thought, not accurate enough to prove the disease was in my lung.

    Yesterday I had to go through another needle lung biopsy, which proved to be a very stressful and traumatic experience. Unlike the first test I had, complications this time. Halfway through the procedure, my vein collapsed, as well as three others and it took a fifth IV catheter to be successful. I have never felt so helpless. There was nothing I could do, and since I was proceeding with the biopsy, my mom couldn't be with me to hold my hand and guide me. I depend on her <u>so</u> much during my tests. She helps me to focus and ignore the pain. I guess she's the inspiration that keeps me strong. Without her, I felt scared and weak and I felt like giving up. Fortunately, after taking three biopsies, I had no collapse of the lung, but a lot of pain, both physical and emotional. I was basically traumatized by the whole experience. Yet, it's funny how sometimes God will send little reminders that he's watching over and won't let anything too dreadful happen to me. A special x-ray technician, named Lynn, spotted me after the procedure and could sense I was down, and to my surprise, on her lunch break, she brought me a card and a stuffed animal. In the card she wrote that she had been thinking and praying *for me. I felt so happy that I cried. It's amazing how something so little can make such a difference. I feel as though God sent her to me to remind me everything was going to be all right.*

Somehow, my life can never be good for very long, because upon my return home, I was disappointed to find that once again Kurt wasn't there for me. In fact, I haven't spoken to him in three days, and he could care less how the test went. It's funny how just on Valentine's Day he claimed he would always be there for me, yet here I am going in for intense lung surgery tomorrow, and he hasn't talked to me, nor does he know. I don't think I'll ever understand what's going through the minds of the friends I have. They must have no conscience to be able to ignore me and my disease for long periods of time. If they only knew what I'm going through and how much they hurt me every time they flake out. Maybe they would think twice. I've decided, after a lot of thinking, to let go of those that continue to hurt me. They will one day realize how much they could have learned and benefited from my loving friendship, and they'll regret everything they did.

Saturday, February 25, 1995

Our consult with Dr. Dan proved to be disheartening. The needle biopsy was not conclusive, so a surgical lung biopsy has been scheduled at 9:00 am this morning. Dr. Howard is a well-respected surgeon, but Amber is anxious about the procedure regardless of his reputation. Her bad experience on Thursday has left her very vulnerable. I underestimated this staging methodology. It is a long and drawn out process of elimination that is necessary for planning what type of treatment will be most effective in ridding her body of the cancer cells.

It is hard to know what to pray for at this point. God's will, I guess. What am I feeling? I must be strong, but at the same time I'm really scared this is only the beginning.

Sunday, February 26, 1995

Amber is resting now. She had such a traumatic two days before. Amazingly, she woke up with a smile, then took her pain med and is now dozing again. I am in awe of her strength.

The procedure finally took place at 1:50; the time neatly etched pictorially in my mind. As I stood next to her gurney in the recovery room, the nurses and anesthesiologist all smiling and making light banter with her and Dr. Howard. He was promising he would do a good job and make the incision small. At the last minute he asked her if she wanted a Hickman, (a central line to the vena cava, a guaranteed vein instead of injecting her each time she has chemotherapy) placed at the same time. She declined saying she would rather take her chances. He was trying to do this while she was going under, but she said, "No way!" Strange how this question was asked so close to actual surgery time.

Tom, Bridgett and I sat in the surgical waiting area. Time passed, and we were not sure what to pray for. I was trying to level out, so I proceeded with crochet work. The games we brought kept the others busy.

At about 3:30, Dr. Howard comes in and the procedure is finally over. He has scooped out the nodule in question and it is Hodgkin's. My prayers have been modified. I now accept the disease in a major organ. Stage IV is now a reality, but at least no laparotomy or thoracotomy is now necessary.

Amber is able to see us in the recovery room, the drugs are apparent in her eyes, tubes in her nose from oxygen being pumped into her "designer" socks for help with circulation during surgery. She looks so small and weak. Her lip is puffed up and she's hooked up to all kinds of beeping things. At this point, I am strong and glad she's OK. She has a tube filled with blood coming out of her chest into a box hooked under the bed. After assessing all this, I concentrate on massaging her feet—giving them a gentle scratch.

I am able to stay with her in her room. The pediatric ward is as warm as a hospital room can be, and the nurses are very special. There isn't much activity in the entire hospital since it's Saturday. Our doctor has no set time frame. In fact, he brought us all ice cream at about nine pm. What a guy!

Amber is so uncomfortable from this tube hanging out. The I.V. inserted on the top of her hand is on the opposite side. The evening is spent watching her in pain, her meds given in shot form, ouch—hold my hand, honey. Let me take away the pain. I love you so much—I hate what's happening to you. I wish it were me instead. Hang on—breathe, and try to think of a pleasant thing—this is impossible to do. For the next several hours, my focus is out of my body— into hers. I don't need sleep or food. I really am so absorbed. The time goes by, different nurses for the duration, but I remain. It's now 8:00 am—I guess I slept a little. Amber is dozing, propped up on her back. I can see by her wincing every movement is painful. Dr. Dan comes in. What a sweetie. He will be our main squeeze from now on. He kisses her on the cheek. Dr. Howard comes in—looking more like a jogger off the streets than a doctor. They both share post-operative concern, one as a surgeon, the other as Amber's oncologist.

Amber has had a chance to eat a little breakfast and go potty—then the decision is made by Dr. Howard to pull the tube out from her lung that has been draining the fluids. Oh boy—I'm not ready for this. Tom and Bridgett are here, but they leave the room. Mentally, I leave too, and my other self is left behind to hold her hand as he gives her a shot to numb the chest area—a whopper—then some Adivan for the pain.

He promises her she won't remember this and then quickly he cuts the sutures and starts pulling out the tube, Amber is beside herself with pain, a long owwwwwww, owwww, owwww, building to a crescendo as she squeezes my hand so tightly it will break soon.... my tears are there...hers too. I can't slip away, must be strong. This is lasting a lifetime...all in about two minutes. I won't forget the agony in her face; too much for one so young. Now it's over. The worst.

　　　Reliving that pain is hard for me, but writing helps to let it go. She is so special. She is my inspiration. Now we must move on... Dr. Dan will see us on Friday. Chemo is the next hurdle we must go over. I'm not sure if I can stay in school. At this point it matters less and less. I got accepted to Cal Poly, that long awaited letter seems like a trivial thing right now. It's only a reminder that life goes on.

Chapter Six

Amber's voice on friends

Tuesday, February 28, 1995

I successfully tackled yet another procedure, and am slowly returning to normal. I'm happy to know that this will be my last. The cancer had progressed to my lungs and chemotherapy will be my form of treatment. I'm having quite a few mixed feelings about all that's happened. I'm glad that all the tests are over, but I'm scared of what's to come.

In my short stay in the hospital, I was surprised to find that Kate and Mona came to visit me and that Kurt sent me flowers. I guess sometimes it takes a serious event to wake people up. Now, three days after surgery, I haven't heard anything from the three of them. Some things never change. I'm trying to accept the fact that I can no longer allow them to change my moods, but it continues to eat at me. If one of them were going through this, I would never treat them like they've treated me. I've mentioned several times to my therapist that I'm considering going into counseling as a career. Knowing how I feel and how hard it is not to have friends to rely on, I feel that in the future, I'm going to help individuals avoid the pain I've been through. There is no hurt worse than feeling alone. For myself, I have to stay positive and happy, so try not to think about each broken promise that arises. I'd rather focus on my loving family and the beauty that surrounds me. I try to imagine myself a few years from now, cured and wiser.

I know that this bumpy road won't last forever. God is watching over me and guiding me. He will never give up on me and he has a particular plan for my future. I don't know why I was chosen to have Hodgkin's, but I do know that it was given to me for a purpose.

Wednesday, March 1, 1995

It may be partially due to the pain meds, but I'm finding myself becoming more and more emotional. At this moment, I feel like crying because I'm sick of all that is happening to me. I talked to an old friend from high school tonight who obviously called because he found out. I was really happy to hear from him, yet I started to think how different my life is than everyone else my age. Here, he is complaining about work, school and how boring life is here and all I can help but wish is that I was in his shoes. I want to be the one complaining once again about finals and work and being away from home. To think I thought my life was shitty in San Diego, what I would give to go back in time.

Today, I spent the day hoping my pain in my back would subside long enough to run some errands with my mother, just so I could get out of the house. Pretty pathetic! The highlight of my day was going to the bank and to get gas. Tomorrow I get to look forward to spending the day alone while my dad's at work, my sister's at school, and my mom is at college. I'm wondering if I'll be able to enjoy the time to myself. Honestly, I'm a little scared. Sometimes I can really get down and frustrated as much as I hate my parents babying me, I really appreciate their company.

The dread of Monday is fastly approaching...my first chemotherapy treatment. I'm so scared. I've been able to put it off this long and now it's becoming a reality. I'm really going to lose my hair! I'm constantly trying to imagine myself looking like Sinead O'Connor. I hope that I don't look too repulsive; then again, who do I have to impress.

Pretty much the only people I see on a regular basis is my family. Maybe that's why God's allowing all of my friends to bail out on me, to save me the embarrassment when I go bald! I guess that's kind of ridiculous, but I know my friends that live here, wouldn't be able to handle it. So, God's doing the both of us a favor.

This battle is one I'm going to have to fight solo. In the end I will be stronger than anyone ever imagined. Positively, I can say that March 1 of 1996 I will have successfully beat this disease and all the heartache that goes along with it!

Thursday, March 2, 1995

Today, I really tried to keep myself busy while everyone was gone. I colored, read, and talked to some friends from USD who surprised me and called. It was up until that point that I was doing well, but hearing them talk about their lives back at school made me a little bit jealous. They claim that life isn't the same without me, and that they miss me, hoping to make me feel good, but I found myself crying after I hung up the phone. I want so much to be able to return and have things be normal again, but obviously it isn't possible.

Spring break is coming up and a bunch of them want to come visit. I want to be excited, yet all I can do is wonder where I'll be in treatment and if I will be losing my hair. I don't think that I'm going to let them come visit, because until I can get used to these changes in my life, I can't be worrying about how other people are going to handle it. There are a lot of unknowns in my life right now. The farthest I can plan ahead is today and it's hard.

I've found that the one I turn to the most is my mom. I swear she is my rock. She's been with me through every procedure, operation, confrontation and social problem. I cry on her shoulder practically every day, and she gives me the will to go on. She is so special to me and I feel blessed to have her. A lot of my friends don't have a close relationship with either of their parents, and I feel very lucky. Through this whole thing, me and my mom have become really close. I find myself talking to her about every feeling and fear I encounter. Without her, my life would really be in pieces. I love her dearly.

Chapter Seven

<u>Help is on the way</u>

Wednesday, March 1, 1995

    I just talked with my mom. She's all packed! Looks like she'll really make it here after all. I can't wait! Amber could use some help right now. Grandma is the ticket. Looks as though my sister, Joan, will not come. Her husband, Don, is having a routine heart biopsy as part of his transplant program. Mom will go from her hometown of Truth or Consequences, NM, to Albuquerque tomorrow and soon will get on the train to come here. This is great. What a shot in the arm for Amber and me. I'm sure Bridgett will benefit from Mom's advice. She listens to her. I know this has been hard for her to see her sister go through so much.

    Amber has been quite tearful lately. Her friends called from San Diego and want to come see her on spring break in a week. She isn't sure if she will feel like having company after her first chemo treatment. She is having so much anxiety. Will she lose her hair? Will she be throwing up? Will she get skinny? Will she be tired? These things set her apart from the "normal" teenager. She has let these worries dominate her day.

    I was gone to school till 4:00 and she was home alone. Now my guilt comes back—should I quit school? She needs me more than ever. I just don't know how much I can help—sometimes I am hovering over her too much. She needs to have some independence, otherwise I'm tempted to do everything for her, tell her what to do, manage her life. She is beginning to isolate herself from the outside world and I have to encourage her to stay busy and maintain her class at the community college and keep in contact with her friends even thought they are "flaky" most of the time. Sandra will be here tonight so that should cheer her up. She brings sunshine into our world and a feeling of how it used to be when Amber was well. It makes me so sad to see her feel so "different." Please hear my prayer and give me some direction to help get her through this huge obstacle in her life. Take away my guilt of being glad she's home, and my mixed emotions about why she's home. I wasn't ready to let her go to college, but I never wished for this.

We saw Dr. Dan yesterday and while waiting for our appointment, a woman named Eadie came in to meet us. Somehow she knew we had an appointment at 4:00 pm and she stopped in purposely to meet us. Her son has Hodgkin's disease and is about Amber's age. What a coincidence, Bridgett knows her from the dance studio—she takes tap there and is a ball of fire, a very positive lady. Amber asked her some questions about the chemo effects her son had. She made it sound not so bad...I felt some relief after talking to her.

Dr. Dan was in a feisty mood— he was really cute. He checked Amber's incisions and pulled off the steri-strips. When he got to her back, one split open and started to bleed. Amber didn't know, just said it stung. I'd put this picture in my brain along with the others— the painful "I wish I could do something" pictures that I can't get out of my head. She has been through so much and I have seen all that she has felt. Her concentration focused on trying not to feel the pain and mine on her. I just kept on talking about trivial things to keep her mind off of it. I must have sounded like an idiot, but it worked.

The information he gave us about chemo is not much different than what we learned reading literature from the American Cancer Society. Bridgett was present for this meeting and could ask questions if she wished. I want her to be more a part of this than she has been up to this point. I hope this will make her more sympathetic to what Amber is going through—not just a bystander. Although Dan didn't go into detail, I know how serious it really is. Bridgett didn't offer much in the way of comments, but I could tell she was paying close attention.

Amber's first treatment will be on Monday at 1:00 pm. The doc says she will feel relief from the itching right away—that will be a blessing for her, I know. I spend nights scratching the bottoms and tops of her feet, her back, her legs, till my arms are tired, then she looks up at me, with her shining blue eyes and her smile of love, and she always says "Thank you, Mom, it feels better now." I put these pictures in my heart and try to recall them when I'm feeling down.

      She wants to get her hair cut today from waist length to above her shoulders. Hair loss seems inevitable, so she wants to take care of some of it now so it won't be such a shock when it begins to fall out. Dr. Dan says it may not happen, that everyone is different, but she's set on the change just in case and even seems excited about it like a rites of passage to move on to the next step of her journey. I often write and think about "we," but it is "she" that is going through the experience and doing a fine job of coping with it. Her therapist is a great help with her techniques of positive imagery through meditative visualization. I'm grateful she can offer that to help her through.

Sunday, March 5, 1995

      Amber got her hair cut to her chin, the shortest she's ever had. Sandra and Kate went with her for support. I bowed out. I never could watch either of my girls get their hair cut. She came home with a big smile looking so cute. It was just what she needed to lift her spirits. Tonight she has a visitor, Todd, her old flame from high school. While he's visiting, I hear her giggle—nervous at first. I'm sitting here thinking negative thoughts about her treatment and how it could possibly make her infertile. I shared my concerns with Tom, and he shakes his head. His solution is that there is always adoption. To me that's not good enough. There's no guarantee either way that the chemo will take away her chance to be a mom, or it won't. I feel like I should have pursued a fertility specialist or something to prevent this from being so final. I am out of_my league here. I will have to talk to Dr. Dan about it. For tonight, I'll try not to think. Tomorrow is the first day of treatment. This week will be a stressful one. I am anxious. I am going to call Eadie and share my fears with her. She has been a good person to talk to. I would like to get Amber and her son, Ray, together so he can share what to expect with her. I'm not going to force it though, that's got to be Amber's idea. She is a little uncomfortable since he's 25 and a guy. I think it would be helpful for her to talk to someone who's been through it already.

Guardian Angel

Guardian Angel by my side
How lovely you must be
To leave your home in heaven
To watch over a child like me
When I'm far away from home
Or having a bad day
I know you will protect me
From harm along the way
How beautiful your face must be
Although I cannot see
Your presence is always of comfort
I know you pray for me
I want so much to thank you
For your loving and caring ways
Never leave me, stay by my side
I hope we'll meet in heaven someday

By Amber Carter, August 1993

Chapter Eight

Infertility, futility, possibility

Sunday, March 5, 1995

     Today, I had a surprise phone call from Todd, who was very concerned about some information he had heard. I thought that by now, he would have heard through the grapevine like everyone else has, but apparently he just found out this morning. In fact, he went straight to the hospital, thinking I was still there. Now I feel totally bad that I didn't tell him myself. He seemed hurt by my actions. I don't know what it is about him, but I think we will always secretly love each other, but, both know it would never work.

     He ended up stopping by my house with a friend to visit for a few hours. We talked and reminisced about old times, and now I find myself wishing there was a small possibility! He had the idea in his mind that I was going to die, and was relieved to find out it was 90% curable. When I told him, he practically looked as if he would cry. I think Todd has changed a lot with time. I honestly felt his concern was genuine.

     The whole situation is ironic because Ms. Sims, my favorite high school teacher, mentioned his name two days ago because she thought I should call him. So, he's been on my mind all weekend. Fate always puzzles me. Things always happen for a reason. I wonder why this happened? All I know is I think I still love him and that really scares me. I start chemotherapy tomorrow at 1:00, and I strangely am excited to get it over with. I'm not even dreading it, which is good because my psyche is up. I feel that the positive thinking is going to do wonders for me!

Monday, March 6, 1995

As I was coming home from taking Bridgett to school I broke down, I just began to cry and it was from my toes—I pulled over and just let it go. I felt much relief, like a dam breaking. When I got home, Amber was awake, shivering in her bed. She said she was nauseous from about 3:00 am on. She was crying and looked pretty helpless. I made her some tea and once she got that down she felt better. I gave her some toast with sugar and cinnamon. This is what God has planned for me—to help my child get through this next step along her path to recovery. The pills she had taken were pre-chemotherapy and were supposed to prevent nausea. What was wrong?

I am now sitting next to my baby while she is getting her first session of chemo. Turns out she was to take only one pill at a time and she took all three at once, hence the opposite effect they were intended for. No damage done, just discomfort. We'll know better next time.

The room is filled with patients, all are at least three times her age. There's a lot of coughing and mumbling and then my eyes focus on one bright, shining face, my angel, Amber. She is so out of place here, she should be shopping or laying out at the beach or attending a class at USD. She shouldn't be here—period!

My latest fear is still there. Should I be doing more to question procedures for my young and still fertile child? Am I not doing enough for her future? Can anything be done? Is it too late? Will I regret this in ten years? That I had not exhausted all possibilities and voiced my opinion and shared my fears and checked on what could be avoided on Amber's behalf? What's the lesser of the two evils? Of course, I'm not stupid. I know she has to get rid of the cancer and chemo seems to be the way to do that, but should we take more precautions for her future that she is not thinking of because she is so young and hasn't considered child bearing as being important? These things race through my mind. I am still consumed with questions about harvesting her eggs and having them frozen so she can create a life with someone she loves that will be one-half Amber. She doesn't want to think about that now and I can understand, but I'm going to do all I can before it is too late to prevent this tragedy. I am determined.

Wednesday, March 8, 1995

Well, today was a pretty good day, unlike my nauseous yesterday. First off, I took my pills wrong and I took 3 anti-nausea pills, which made me have muscle spasms and nervousness. Now I know I only take those when needed. Me and my mom are learning the hard way

:) Nonetheless, today I woke up in a good mood and decided that this evening would be a country western night. I've been bummed enough about Kurt, so I told Hillary I would double date with this guy Anthony. So, my plans were made for the evening after my night class. The night turned out kind of depressing. Once again, I was thinking of Kurt, hoping he would show up, but only found that his friends showed, which automatically makes me assume he's avoiding me. Once again, I don't get it. I'm really sick of these games he plays, and have vowed that I will care no more for him. He can come running to me when he realizes what he's lost!

On a good note, I also found out today that if I, by chance, become infertile due to the chemo, my sister can donate eggs to me. We have the same genetic make up, and with today's technology, it has been done before. So, one of my biggest concerns is somewhat calmed. I hope it won't result in that, but at least there's hope :)

Monday, March 13th

I finished my first cycle of chemotherapy today. From here, I don't have a pretty pathway planned, but at least so far I've tolerated the treatment well. Dr. Dan is impressed how well I've handled it to this point, which makes me feel good. I'm finally not sad about the hair thing. I think the anticipation will be the worst, along with the actual act of losing it. But, I really feel that this is going to happen for a reason. If I can love myself without hair, I'll be able to love myself no matter what. Maybe this is what it will take for me to improve my low self-esteem.

My spiritual side has been strengthened so much in the past two months. Besides my family, my faith has been what's pulled me through accepting the disease, giving me courage to follow through with procedures, to deal with my fears, accept lost friends and push towards remission with a positive attitude. Without faith, none of this would be possible.

These events that are happening to me are all happening for a reason. It's not my job to figure out why, but, rather to take each obstacle and deal with it. In the end, I know that this will grant me infinite wisdom and insight.

The Beach

The powerful waves crash against the sandy beach. Seagulls take flight in fear of the approaching storm. Tourists scurry in all directions to take shelter in their vehicles. Suddenly, all is vacant at the once crowded beach.

Out of nowhere a stranger approaches and stares out into one of the wonders of nature, the deep blue ocean. It amazes him that something so beautiful could possess such power. He stares out into the deep blue and reflects on all of the problems in his life. They all seem so small compared to the ocean that stretches as far as he can see. He leaves with a different outlook on life.

By Amber Carter 1993

Chapter Nine

<u>Angels of hope</u>

Thursday, March 9, 1995

So much has happened, I'm busting with news. Upon contacting the American Cancer Society, I was given the opportunity to talk with Helen, who is an oncology nurse. After explaining Amber's dilemma, she shed much light on the subject of infertility due to chemotherapy. Since Amber has a sister, there can be an egg transfer from her to a dish and fertilized with sperm and placed in Amber. In other words, Bridgett's eggs would be used to solve the possibility of Amber becoming infertile. Because they have similar genetics, it will be close to what Amber produces for herself. What an absolute relief this is for me! Helen is my Angel of Hope.

We are sitting in the waiting area for Amber's second treatment and a visit with the doc. There are a few here before us. Hurry and wait is the regular procedure. So, I have some time to jot down my thoughts. This weekend was stormy in more ways than the weather. Bridgett went out on Friday night, against my better judgment. That same night we had quite a rainstorm and flooding in the area. She begged her dad and I to go out on a double date. We let her go with the stipulation she call us when she reached her friend's house.

By 11:30 pm she still had not called. With one daughter home sick from chemotherapy, my nerves were already rattled. Finally, I called her myself at her friends' house. She gave me an excuse of being stuck in the mud of their driveway all night. Could I believe her? My nerves were frazzled. She was ordered home and grounded for the remainder of the weekend for not calling us. That went over like a lead balloon.

Tom and I went to our Marriage Encounter Circle and got out a lot of feelings about Amber's illness and our teenage rebellious Bridgett. When we got home, Amber had been left alone all day while Bridgett went shopping. We had counted on her staying home with her sister and helping her out. The effects of the first session of chemo had left Amber quite ill. I just didn't understand how Bridgett could have left her in that condition.

There was no way to resolve this conflict. Bridgett had become completely defensive. The weekend ended with her refusal to attend church with the family. The one saving grace was the news that my mother is coming to visit us in a couple of weeks and my sister Judy will accompany her on the train.

Thursday, March 16, 1995

My mom is finally here and my sister, Judy, too. They brought the New Mexico sunshine with them. It's an adjustment with two extra adults in this small house, but its OK with me. It has been hectic the last two days, but now I'm finished with school and it's going to be better.

Amber is doing so well. She won't have chemo for another couple weeks. We expected her to be sick, but she had only some night sweats and she says she is a little more tired. I'm so grateful. She expects to lose all her hair now, but I'm holding onto the hope that it won't happen. So far, her side effects have been mild and the doc is very pleased. The lump in her neck has been reduced in size and her itching is gone. This is the answer to many, many prayers. I called my brother, John, and his wife Camille to tell them how well she is doing. Camille has been sending daily letters to Amber. They were elated to hear of Amber's progress. The prayers are working.

Mom and Judy have been her since Tuesday and we've done some shopping, some whale watching and have done a lot of talking. Mom is obsessed with pulling out all the weeds in the garden, so she's been pretty busy. After the rain, the flowerbeds are covered with them. My husband is being patient with two extra females in the house. He's outnumbered five to one. His lack of privacy is an issue, but he's doing ok for the most part.

Amber is still amazing me. She has a good appetite, not nauseous at all, even went out with her friends to a party last night. Her smile has been infectious to all around her.

Tuesday, March 21, 1995

Amber is doing great! She hasn't lost any hair, hasn't been sick or overly tired. She just has some days that are slightly better than others. Her appetite is good, too. She took her last Predinasone yesterday, now will be off all meds for two more weeks. The blood draw went well yesterday. The lab tech got a vein in the first poke. Her doc has to monitor the white and red cell count and platelets. Sometimes a blood transfusion is necessary if those counts are low due to the chemotherapy killing the good cells off as well as the cancer cells. She hasn't had that happen yet, and we'll cross that bridge together if we come to it. She has been in good spirits knowing she has a break for two weeks.

Meanwhile, my mom is bringing happiness into our house. She is a ball of fire and I get tired just watching her. Making dinner, doing laundry, pulling weeds. I practically have to tie her down. We tease her with the name "the energizer bunny that keeps going and going." She has lots of positive vibes surrounding her and it filters out to us all. Judy went back yesterday. Amber and I drove her to the bus in Goleta so she could catch the shuttle that will take her to L.A. to catch her plane.

Wednesday, March 22, 1995

I successfully completed my first cycle of chemotherapy. So far, I haven't lost my hair. I wake up every morning anticipating finding it gone, but it's still there. Slowly, my energy level has built back up. I almost feel "normal."

I went country dancing tonight and Kurt was there. I hate that we aren't talking and I felt weird the whole night. Until I, of course, initiated a conversation with him. Things were really weird at first, but then he asked me to dance and I felt myself drift into the past. I can't help it, I feel so natural with him. It was all I could do to fight the urge to kiss him when we were slow dancing, but I managed to play it as friends. Like I had guessed, he was mad about my telling Kate about his experimentation with crank. I knew when I told her that I was wrong, but in a way I was trying to hurt him like he's hurt me. Anyway, we decided to be friends again and we'll see how it works out. Anything's better than being enemies. Who knows, maybe someday he'll turn out to be the one, but for now I have to just let go. Luckily, Kate has taken his place and become a dependable friend once again. As strong as I believe myself to be, I still am needy of a companion and I'm glad she's there for me.

God has a way of allowing things to work out. Everything in his world happens for a reason. Knowing this has helped me survive the past few months. This is where my true faith in him is tested.

"If you love something very much,

Let it go free...

If it doesn't come back

It wasn't meant to be...

If it does, love it

Forever..."

(My quote for the evening) :)

Thursday, March 23, 1995

 I just finished writing a letter to Dr. Steward to send with our co-pay. I wanted to tell him he had a tough job to do, telling Amber and I on that fateful night that she had cancer. Even though it must have been so hard for him, he did handle it well. I wonder what he was thinking? Did we react as he thought we would? Did he leave us alone and then go out in the hall and hit something because of the unfairness of it all? Did he already know the long road ahead of us, and the staging process she would have to endure? If there was a movie being done about that night, and they could cut away and show his reactions, what would they have been? I wonder. I know the memory is forever deeply etched in my mind: the pain on Amber's face when she looked into my eyes with tears and said to me "I don't want to die!" Oh.... I can't even let that creep out of my subconscious today; I will certainly be a gonner. So, try to think of the pleasant things of today. Amber is feeling great—no treatments or pills for one more week. She went to Santa Barbara to visit Abby and have some fun. I'm amazed at her. She has been drinking the special herbal tea that Sandra's mother gave her, and it seems to be giving her energy. That, combined with her being between chemo cycles, is probably the reason she is doing so well. She is examining her hair loss each morning, and looks a little panicked, and then tries to continue on with her day. I think if it ever goes, she will accept it—this is the next dilemma then that should be all of the "surprises." I know she still hopes to be the one that doesn't lose hair with chemotherapy.

 Meantime, I am thoroughly enjoying my mom being here. We went to yard sales today and had fun. She is a trip. She is filled with so much energy and stamina. I am very blessed she came to stay with us.

Chapter Nine

<u>Golden hair</u>

Sunday, March 26, 1995

    Today was a difficult day...I have started to lose my hair. As much as I had hoped I would be the exception to the rule, the inevitable has come. I thought that I had mentally prepared myself, but I don't think anyone can realize what it is like until it happens. I can't even run my fingers through my hair without tangling 10-15 hairs around my fingers. Unlike regular hair loss, it is never ending. I decided to put it back in a ponytail so I don't have to deal with it falling out and sticking to my clothes. At least I cut my long hair before this happened. I can't imagine having long hairs tangled in my fingers and brush. I have an urge just to buzz it all off so I don't have to go through weeks of hair loss, but I don't have the guts. Who knows what the best way to handle this is?!?

    I went to visit my friend from USD this weekend in Santa Barbara. Abby came down (from college) as sort of a surprise. I haven't seen her in 2 months. Our visit at first was good and we decided to go to a movie with her parents, and up until this point, I was enjoying my visit. Then she took me to a friend of hers house who was having a party. She met up with her high school buddies who were also home from college. They reminisced and shared college stories for the whole night, while the people surrounding were drinking and smoking and having a good time. I really felt outside of it all. I'm not able to experience the same carefree fun that most people my age are. I found as my spirits dropped, so did my feeling of wellness. I no longer felt disease-free as I had the week before. We ended up leaving at 11:30 and went back to her house. I left Santa Barbara today feeling negative and down. I returned to find my hair falling out. Just when I think I'm doing good, something happens to remind me I'm different, and will be forever.

Wednesday, March 29, 1995

Amber's hair is really falling out now. She goes in and out of emotions about it. Mostly, she can't style it because she says the hair just hangs loosely afterwards—so she has taken to wearing a ponytail snug at the base of her head. Her dad wanted to show her that people don't change just because they don't have hair, so he had me buzz his head. How can he know the difference of a girl in her teens, watching her crowning glory fall away before her very eyes? It was a valiant effort on his part, but it still only lessens the emotions tied in with her personal dilemma. I see her wanting to isolate from her peers. She doesn't want to go to the Grad with her hair "like that." I can talk until I'm blue about beauty being on the inside, she just says, "I know, but..."

So, day-to-day we go. Sandra comes into town today. Maybe she can cheer her up like only another teen (best buddy) can do.

The tea seems to help Amber's energy level. It's a positive approach that gives her and Grandma something to do to alleviate her side effects of the chemo. Her appetite is still good, and some days I have trouble believing she's sick at all. Then, I see the trash can filled with hair, and I know this is for real. She also has pains in her chest from the tumor there that is the size of her fist. That's real, too.

Wednesday, March 29, 1995

It's Wednesday, and once again the Grad was on. Only, this time Sandra was here and my buddy and I had a great time. Sometimes I look at her and am <u>so jealous.</u> She's skinny, beautiful and carefree. She's able to go out and party, experience college and so all the things I can't and won't be able to do for a long time. She came home from Lake Havasu, AZ, for their spring break with so many raging stories to tell. It took an hour and a half to explain it all. While in one week, I've done enough to take up about five minutes of explaining. I know that there is a reason for what I am going through, but I just feel so rejected right now and I need someone and of course I'm after what I can't have. That's the way it works!

I refuse to let myself be depressed, so enough about Kurt...My week of no drugs or food restrictions is coming to a close. I'm so bummed. :(I've enjoyed eating cheese and sour cream and bananas I've been deprived of for three weeks. Now I get to start the sequence all over again on Monday. I'm thrilled!!! At least I have 1 behind my belt, now only five more (I pray!)

Chapter Ten

<u>Could this be a miracle?</u>

Wednesday, April 5, 1995

Tom and I went to the beach alone and we talked for a while. I felt the tension ease after that. Monday brought such good news to us all. Amber's x-ray taken on Sunday was compared to the one taken after her biopsy in January. The current one shows no big mass in her chest!! In fact, Dr. Dan says she is as clean as a whistle! How can that be? She has had only one chemo treatment. Well, I say it's the power of prayer. This is as close to a miracle as I'll ever see!

At first, Amber and I were in shock about the news. Then as it sunk in, we rejoiced! We were able to give our loved ones and friends some good news! She will still have to have five more sessions of therapy, but she feels great! No ill affects so far, no nausea or loss of appetite. In fact, she gained 2 pounds since her last appointment. Of course, she's upset about gaining weight, but I am elated. I thought I'd be watching her dwindle to nothing from being unable to eat. Her hair is still falling out, but she got her wig yesterday, and aside from it having bangs, it looks like her own hair.

Amber and I had our ballet mid-term yesterday. She was right next to me and had no problem doing the class. I am amazed at her strength. Against the odds, she is recovering each session of chemo with no ill side effects to speak of.

I am so grateful to God for her progress. My heart fills with love each time I think of it. We have come so far within such a short time. I have prayed for this day. I have hope.

Friday, April 7, 1995
        Amber and I performed a dance we created together last night at the college. We both wore matching scarves and ballet skirts. The music was "The Friendship Song" from the movie Beaches. We are truly friends in every sense of the word. I feel such a bond between us now—we have been through hell together, and now see the light on the other side. I still know she must individuate from me, but last night, we were in sync as the audience watched us perform together. Her dad, sister and grandma were there watching. When I look at her, I see only beauty, inside and out. I am proud to be her mother and friend. I am grateful God gave me the strength to endure watching her pain and her victories over the cancer. Recovery is such a shallow, empty word. There is so much more that goes into it, the mental, as well as the physical. It's a major shot of reality and a constant reminder of how fragile our lives are.

April 1995
        So much for me writing as much as I said I would. I can't even begin to explain everything that has happened to me. I guess I shouldn't say to me, but to my sister. She was diagnosed with Hodgkin's disease, which is a type of cancer.
        I still remember the day I found out. My mom was picking me up from Karen's house and she told me the news. We all cried and cried. I didn't really know what the heck to do. To make a long dramatic story short she had test after test; operations which were scary; and is now going through chemotherapy. She lost her hair and that was hard to get used to. It still is hard to look at her.
        I guess why I really wanted to write is because I'm having some odd feelings. I know I can't be jealous that my mom is paying a lot of attention to Amber. I know my sister needs it. It's just I felt that before the "NEWS" my mom and I had a really good relationship going. I felt close to her and it was really nice. Now, all we do is fight and argue. We never talk or she never is there anymore. I mean she is, but she isn't. Her mind is always on Amber. I guess I am jealous, although I could never admit it to anyone else, but I just feel <u>alone</u> and it makes me really sad.   BC

Tuesday, April 8, 1995
        Well, I started my second cycle of chemo on Monday, and was given some wonderful news for a change. My latest chest x-ray was compared to that before treatment, and miraculously revealed no sign of cancer. The news was shocking. To think I was going to be happy

with the mass shrinking a millimeter and come to find out it disappeared as easily as it appeared. Everyone I've told is amazed and most everyone has cried, but I'm afraid to get too excited because I fear that it will return. I don't want to jinx what has happened, but I just feel so lucky. First of all, I haven't had any dramatic side effects that I heard so much about (besides the hair thing) and now with only one month of therapy, I'm practically cured. It's hard to look back and think how much I've been through up until this point. I have been through tests, operations, blood samples, x-rays, biopsies, IV's, hair loss, weight gain, friend loss, love loss and now this disease has just packed up and left, leaving me with four more months of hell to go through. (Being that six cycles of chemo is the minimum.) So, yes, I am happy, but I would have much rather not had it at all.

When I shared this news with Todd, his reaction was like everyone else's... He was excited and insisted on taking me to a movie to celebrate, but he couldn't do it Tuesday, had class on Wednesday, his birthday was on Thursday, so Friday was the best bet. "I'll call you Thursday and let you know what time." Well, today is Friday, and he never called. That's the story of my life. Just what I wanted, another flaky friend to make a promise he knew he wouldn't keep. Get real, why would he want to take out an ex-girlfriend with cancer to a movie on a Friday night. I'm sure that he would have had to miss out on some really important party or something. Oh well... once again, c'est la vie! For now, I'm not meant to have a social life. I swear, if these so-called friends of mine would put themselves in my shoes for about a day and had to put up with the shit I have to and get let down by the ones who "claim" they care, they wouldn't be able to last an hour. There is not one friend of mine whom I feel could handle this disease and all that it comes with the way I have, and I'm damn proud of it. One day I'm going to write a book about this whole trauma and these friends of mine are going to cry knowing they could have helped make things a lot easier on me and maybe, just maybe I'll help friends like mine who know of someone with cancer not make the same mistakes!

Daddy's Girl

He cares so much
it hurts inside
The pain is deep
too deep to hide

He tries to speak
chokes up instead
Then gently tears
roll from his head

But work he must
his heart s heavy
Provide for us
secure and steady

One foot steps
in front of the other
A minute crawls by
and then another

But thoughts remain
through out his day
"God, make her well
I pray, I pray"

To Tom
From Janine
1996

Chapter Eleven

<u>Life goes on</u>

Sunday, April 9, 1995

Our little Bridgett tried out for Varsity Cheerleader today and didn't make it. My poor baby girl's heart is broken. She came out crying after the tryouts, and so I knew she wasn't confident enough of the job she had done. I almost can't believe it. She looked good here at home practicing, even though she had waited until the last minute to create her cheer. She and Amber were working on it and it was good seeing them dancing together again. Amber wasn't feeling so hot, and this helped get her off the couch for a while.

I guess there is some lesson God wishes Bridgett to learn from this. My heart hurts for her; she has to face her friends feeling like a failure. I know she is not, but she feels pretty low right now. Nothing I can say or do will make her feel better. She has to feel this way for a while I guess. I just don't want her to hate school any more than she does already. My prayer is that she sees the humbling experience as a stepping-stone and tries harder when she performs the next time. I still think she has what it takes to and do anything she puts her mind to.

Monday, April 8, 1995

Finished up my Prednisone today, and am happy to look forward to two weeks before my next cycle. I despise Prednisone. I've gained about seven pounds since I started therapy and hate every one of them. Not only do I have to be bald, but fat as well. The doctor feels it's good that I've gained, but I can't force myself to look at it in a positive sense. At least I don't have anyone seeing me naked, then I would really be self conscious.

      I had my first visitors this past Thursday. Abby and Pete from USD. I dreaded it all week, because no one except my family had seen me without hair. Sure enough, Abby wanted to see me without my scarf, but I refused. It's funny how some people really don't think before they act. I immediately felt abnormal once again. I can't wait until this treatment is over. Abby's visit was fortunately a short one, and disappointing for her because she couldn't return to USD to tell of my baldhead. Luckily, Sandra came home for Easter weekend. It's amazing how much closer I am to her. Never once did I feel ashamed of what I looked like. In fact, having her here for the weekend improved my self-image slightly. Just knowing that I'll always have her as my best friend made things a little better. We're going to Disneyland in about a week, so now I have something to look forward to! It makes the time pass quickly.

      Todd finally called a week after he claimed he would, which is pretty typical of the old him. I wasn't home and I didn't return his call. I feel like there is no point. I don't want to keep in touch with someone who flakes. If I wanted that I would still be talking to Kurt!!! So, I've let that one go as well. I find that I'm a loner these days. I have no desire to put effort into one-way friendships. I would rather be alone than be continually hurt. I reminisce of yesterdays and high school, and envy how simple it was and how many "friends" I had. It's sad to think that those pages of time are written and turned, but at least I have the memories.

Monday, April 10, 1995

      Amber has felt very tired and more nauseous this week after her second cycle of chemotherapy. On Wednesday she never left the couch and I finally resorted to a liquid supplement in a malt just to get some nourishment into her. She was also quite anxious about her friends from USD coming to visit her on Thursday. The fears of them seeing her without hair were real. She looks radiant with her silk scarf neatly pulled flat over her forehead and we have mastered the bouffant bow tucked neatly back at the base of her neck. Her fair complexion and large blue eyes set off the look of one who had chosen to wear a scarf as a fashion statement rather than a balding cancer patient hiding the fact.

      When the dreaded visiting hour finally came, Amber plastered a smile on her face, opened the door and greeted her company with all the grace and courage of a princess greeting her peers.

      They sat and visited sharing stories of their days at the dorm and all the antics of their college semester together. Then Abby had the nerve to ask Amber to take off her scarf so she could see her bald head. The fear she had worked so hard to overcome came back at that one ugly moment. I could see the damage it had done to her self confidence and I held my breath knowing I would be there to pick up the pieces after they left. But, Amber was able to shake it off. She is learning how to dodge the spears of those with no sense of compassion. Blessed be those that suffer the abuse of others.

Meanwhile, my mom is busy canning Amber's tea, and doing laundry. She is the Energizer Bunny! I will miss her a lot when she goes back home. It's been great having her here. Now, we'll get back to our little family unit. It seems like she just got here, but that was a month ago. She will be 75 years old this month, she doesn't act it. I'm grateful to spend time with her; our lives went on, and we didn't have to entertain her. She saw us at our best and at our worst. She will have lots of stories to tell the family back home. It will be a long while before I get to see her again. We won't be going to Albuquerque this summer. Amber will be going through treatments until August. Even though the scans show shrinkage of the tumors, there is a minimum amount of six cycles Dr. Dan says she has to go through before she "graduates." Maybe we can take a cruise or something to celebrate her final treatment. It's nice to look to the future with hope of good things.

Saturday, April 15, 1995

We celebrated Tom's birthday in grand style! Grandma bought Chinese food for all! After cake and ice cream and opening presents, Amber, Sandra, and Bridgett scrambled for the door to go out to have some fun. Bridgett went to a sleepover at a friends house (she's finally getting over her semi-isolation after not making cheerleader) and Amber and her best buddy were off to get a movie and watch it at Sandra's house and then soak in the hot tub until they get wrinkled up. I am grateful for the busy-ness, glad my girls have friends to be with. This has been a hard week to get through and we all deserve a break.

Chapter Twelve

Grandma's departure

Tuesday, April 18, 1995

Sitting here eating a muffin, it's quiet. Mom left on the train yesterday and arrives in Albuquerque around 2:00 pm today. I feel some loneliness today. I miss her smiling face. Mom is a constant in my life. She gives me strength. She's not very good at sharing her feelings, and we didn't have any of those "comfort crying" shared moments. She did almost cry once, when Amber was upset about losing her hair. But, she quickly left the room. Anyway, we did have some meaningful chats at the table about life and its stresses and unfairness.

It's now Tuesday night, and Mom got home all right. She is so spunky. A little old man she met on the train helped her with her bags when it was time to transfer to the next train. I hope I'm as spry at 75 !! I miss her. She gave as much as she was capable of. I'm glad she came out here to see where we live and what we do and how well Amber is doing and how up and down she can be. It's hard to convey this to anyone until they live here and experience it for themselves. It's just our life, I guess.

Amber has a scratchy throat tonight. I worry about her. I'll call Dr. Dan in the morning. She sometimes has this illusion that she's like everyone else. Just like this weekend, when she lost a filling and thought she could just get it fixed—no can do—

have to consult with Dr. Dan first. If her blood work is ok, then it's all right to proceed, if not, then no work can be done on her teeth. It so happens that her white cells are up, so she's OK. Everything must go through Dr. Dan first. I can't blame her for wanting to be "normal, "but she won't be for a long time. Even after chemotherapy is over, she'll have to have regular blood work done and x-rays for the next few years. I really don't know all the ramifications, but she's hardly like most kids her age. This is going to change her life forever. I can't get so heavy. We've got a lot to be thankful for. The progress and her prognosis is good for a cure. One day at a time. Talk it and believe it, Janine!

Wednesday, April 19, 1995

Boy—-if anyone knows how to push buttons, it's Bridgett. I don't know what caused her bad day, but she didn't come to discuss it with me. Her way of asking permission has become more like a statement of what she is planning, and then she climbs down my throat when I ask for details. "What camp out with Hilary? You want to stay Friday night at Lopez Lake, then who's bringing you to work at 9:30 am on Saturday from there? What performance on Saturday in Santa Maria? Who is taking you there?" By the time we got home from me carting her to the dance studio for a class, we were in full combat. I was tempted to kick her out of the car and have her walk home—if it hadn't been dark, I would have done it.

I'm sure this bad day had something to do with her friend that made cheerleader giving her a ride today. Seems like when Amber is happy doing something (she went to Disneyland with the Sandra and her parents, their treat to her) Bridgett is in the dumps. She is not a happy child. She has great highs, usually from a boy's attention, and great lows, usually from lack of the above. Her moods are a roller coaster, and I have to get off the ride. I'm hanging on for dear life and I just need to bail out and walk awhile.

Friday, April 21, 1995

*It's a Friday night, and once again I stayed home with the fam and watched a rented movie. No one called to invite me out, in fact no one called at all. It's funny how when I was away at college, my homecoming was such a big deal. I would have to turn down plans in order to spend time with my family and people would tell me how much they missed me and how they wished I hadn't gone away. Now…I've been home for four months, and really have *0* friends to speak of. Kate calls every now and then, but the only time we go out is when Sandra's in town. Not once has she suggested we do something together. Hillary hasn't called in a couple weeks. I guess they all think I enjoy always being at home watching TV and hanging out with my family. But, to be truthful, I would rather have my family with me, then have* shitty friends with me. I just wish, for a moment, I could feel "normal." And I could go out without the constant reminder that I'm different. "I'm sick of being sick!!" Now, I know what this quote really feels like. At the rate I'm going, before long I'm going to be a recluse. You know it's gotten bad when you look forward to running errands with your mom just so you have something to do.

I feel selfish to be feeling sorry for myself, considering I've been given a second chance to live, but I really hate the way life is right now. I hate being on hold while everyone else's moves on. I hate that I have to hide in my room when my sisters' friends come over, because I'm too embarrassed of my scraggly head. I hate the feeling of nervousness when someone comes to the door and I secretly hope it's not for me. I hate that Kurt doesn't give a damn how I'm doing as well as the rest of my so-called local friends. I hate my scratchy wig, and the way it looks like a helmet on me with bushy bangs. I hate my cheesy thighs and fat rolls. And with all this in mind I manage to have a smile on my face each and every day. Not many could do it.

Chapter Thirteen

<u>Dawn of acceptance</u>

Monday, May 8, 1995

It's been a while since I wrote last, but as time progresses, I feel like doing less and less. My energy level is pretty low this third cycle. At least I can say it's half way over. Time has really started to help my insecurities of no hair and weight gain. (Not that I like either, but have rather accepted it.) I try to get out in public more. I helped as an Alumni choreographer for the finale of Dance Kaleidoscope at Arroyo Grande High School a couple of weeks ago and had fun, with the exception of a rude girl named Carly who thought it would be wise to comment on my "nice bandana!" Let's just say this sarcastic remark almost stopped me from returning the next day. Sometimes, high school kids can be <u>so</u> cruel. Anyway, I did return in spite of embarrassment, and took a huge step for me. The girl, needless to say, feels like shit now because my sister had a friend inform her that I have cancer and this was why I felt a need for a "bandana." I hope that possibly might have taught her a lesson for the future and saved someone else's feelings.

Other outings I have made in a scarf are, Disneyland, Dance Kaleidoscope, The Secret Garden play, and a mall performance done by my sister. I basically feel more honest and natural not pretending to have hair. My biggest public appearance happened today. KSBY Channel 6 News interviewed me for Nurse Awareness Week. Recommended by Dr. Dan's office for an interview, I was asked to tell how nurses have impacted my life through out my ordeal. The interview took place this morning during therapy. They taped me while getting my IV, as well as my drugs. My disease is no longer a secret to anyone. My intention is to hopefully help others in my position and shed some hope. I left the office feeling positive, and far from ashamed.

I recently had Kurt's mom come up to me at church to ask how I was feeling and give her an update. I was touched, yet hurt that Kurt hasn't even bothered to ask. She admitted Kurt hadn't talked to me in a "couple of weeks" so she wanted to ask herself. I corrected her by adding it had been a couple of months, and told her my good news. She was thrilled and according to word of mouth, Kurt is mad because she confronted him about ditching me as a friend. All I have to say is "guilty conscience" once again. He told Hillary that he wants to call now that things are all right. Well, I say forget it!! Forgiveness is something each and every one of my flaky friends are going to have to <u>slowly</u> earn or not receive!

Wednesday, May 10, 1995

It seems like our lives have been whipped up in a tornado funnel and we are all swirling around in the debris. Bridgett is desperately trying to individuate herself in the midst of our family crises. Amber is in the most threatening ordeal of her life: cancer. Tom is suffering with the pressures of financial struggles and the unending stream of medical expenses, trips, and his own inability to fix everything and make it all better. This huge problem has gripped us all by the neck and I am just trying to rescue our family from the evil that has crept into our lives. United we stand, divided we fall. This shall be our mantra.

I have had some time to reflect back on the early days of Amber's diagnosis and the entire staging process. Tears are still falling and some days it's hard to think of anything else. She is in her third cycle of chemo and even though her side effects are minimal, I still know there is a battle being fought and her body is the battlefield. She has been very tired and listless the past couple of days. Her emotions also are dictated by the meds she is on. The Prednisone has increased her appetite, and contrary to what I thought would happen, she is eating very well, so well that she's gained ten pounds. This is highly unusual according to the literature on chemotherapy side effects. Of course, she is probably pacifying herself by eating, not uncommon for her to do. Also not uncommon to be stressed about it and how this makes her look. I have given my lecture on how this is a good thing for her body to have the extra calories to help fight the effects of chemo and fight any infection that may come up as a result of a low immune system. She is stubborn and calls herself fat. Why is it always something? She can't be satisfied that she is successfully fighting cancer in her body. I have to accept her level of maturity. She is a teenager, after all. What could be worse than gaining ten pounds and losing your hair? She has resigned herself to accept the way she has to look for now, and once her treatments are finished, the weight will come off.

On a brighter note, we received free tickets from the American Cancer Society to go to Great America, an amusement park in the San Francisco area. I am excited to get away from here and do something fun. Now we just need to juggle the bills so we can afford the hotel, meals, etc. It will be worth the effort. That's what charge cards are for, right?

Amber was on the news last night doing an interview about the importance of nurses. I guess it's Nurse Week or something. She was interviewed at Dr. Dan's office and she did a fantastic job. She looked so pretty and was very articulate. We do love the nurses there. They are always upbeat, compassionate, and caring. I wouldn't be able to do their job. Taking care of my baby is one thing, but to care for patients when some of them are terminal must be excruciating. They have to mix and administer the poisonous drugs that kill human cells. Sometimes the veins don't cooperate and the pressure of being successful in the first poke is always there. I have great admiration for all of them.

Chapter Fourteen

Life as we know it

Monday, May 18, 1995

Great America was a blast, the barbeque was nice, and I even got a corsage for Mother's Day. We had our picture taken as a family. Professional pictures haven't been too popular with Amber since she started losing her hair, but she was willing to pose with us for the memory. We stayed at a nice hotel on Saturday and the girls and Tom swam while I soaked in the Jacuzzi. I could hear them playing Marco Polo, just like when they were little. Daddy was always there to have fun with. He's quite a guy.

We left on Sunday in a rainstorm and journeyed home. On the way we played games in the car and enjoyed each other's company. The relaxation and laughter was much needed for all of us. It was a day to remember.

While we were at the amusement park, Amber saw a small girl with cancer who wasn't afraid to go "au natural" and let her bald head be uncovered. It gave her the courage to have her head buzzed. I volunteered to do the deed, putting my heart in my pocket until I could pull it out later and cry my eyes out. There I was, holding a pair of shears, and this time I couldn't avoid it. She is finally at a stage of acceptance of her appearance and even let two of Bridgett's friends see her without her scarf on. That took courage. I am very proud of her. Always.

Since we've been home, Amber helped me with my homework for the early childhood class I am taking. I had to make a box of activities for certain age groups. After that is done and turned in, I have two finals left, and then the semester is over. Thank goodness. I will be elated when this time next week is here. It will be a relief. It hasn't been easy staying in school while Amber is having chemo. I want to be with her as much as I possibly can. Some days I wish I could have a clone so I could be in both places at the same time. She depends on me. I want her to. Our lives are joined by the love we have for each other.

Meanwhile, we are busy preparing for Bridgett's junior prom. She has her dress already. It is a long slinky black one, but very appropriate for her age. She looks quite grown up in it, has the curves, but alas, no boobs. She makes up for those with her smile, and what nature didn't provide, a little padding does wonders. I won't be getting much sleep on Saturday night. We've set curfew at two a.m. I hope everything goes ok, and she has fun. I remember my proms; I loved getting ready for them.

Saturday, May 22, 1995

When Bridgett remembers her Junior Prom, I hope she only re-creates the good parts. It went something like this:

"I just won't help you then," Amber tearfully stomped out of the bedroom.

"What got into her?" Haley quipped.

"She's just in a bad place right now. My sister has lost her friends, her hair, and her hope of ever being normal again." Bridgett answered, pre-occupied with a stubborn curl.

"I don't understand. What happened to all of them?"

"She thought she had some, but one by one they have flaked out on her. I don't understand it either. Just when she needs someone to comfort her, they are dumping her like a bad habit. I do know that I'm sick of her being sick. It just bugs sometimes."

I couldn't help overhearing this dialogue. My heart was in my throat, but I dared not to get caught eavesdropping for fear of repercussions later for butting in. There are some things your children have to work out for themselves, and no matter how much I wanted to console Amber, and defend her mood, I knew I had to turn on my heel and walk away from it. I hated to admit it, but when Amber would get into this self-pity mode, I just wanted to scream myself. I was at the point of knocking their heads together when Hilary finally left, and Amber came out of hiding. She continued to help Bridgett get ready for her big night, vacillating between being insecure and vulnerable one minute to bitchy and self-pitying the next. Bridgett didn't patronize her. She just kept treating her like a big sister, albeit a bit tearful, and she was incredulous of the cruelties of Amber's flaky friendships.

"Your friends are just a bunch of jerks. Especially Kate. She had the nerve to tell you about the big party on Saturday that you weren't invited to." Bridgett spat the words out. "If she were my friend I'd tell her where to go."

At least she was on her side and she said what we all were thinking. That's Bridgett.

"And why does Todd call you up and promise to take you to a movie, then never calls? He has shit for brains, if you ask me."

"I don't know, Bridgie, I just know I wanted to help you get ready and Haley was taking my place. I can't talk to you about the other stuff now." Amber put up the fences.

At that point, I had the biggest desire to go to her, but I had to remind Bridgett of the time and make the house presentable for picture taking. She only had a half-hour before her date, just a friend named Joey, was to pick her up in the limo. The crisis had passed and Cinderella was ready for the ball.

In retrospect, I had to pat myself on the back for not becoming the referee between my girls. I had climbed into that role too many times, and come out the only loser. With Amber being so moody, I had tried to rescue her many times by finding fault with her sister to compensate for the bad hand she'd been dealt. After all, hadn't she been through the absolute worst in the last four months? Along with the diagnosis she had been sentenced to a life of physical pain, change and a constant fear of dying. She had gone from a responsible 18 year old in college with a job, classes, and new friends to an overweight, baldheaded, insecure cancer patient who had been abandoned by longtime friends and was totally dependent on her mom and dad for everything, including friendship. I kept these things to myself, wrote them down, cried and tried to let it go. I had many sleepless nights trying to make sense of it all. I never did. Sleep, that is, or make sense of it.

Wednesday, May 24, 1995

Tonight, I went out dancing for the first time in over two months. I forced myself to accept an invitation from Hilda to go to the Graduate (a nightclub for teens). After days of stressing over what I was going to wear on my buzzed head, I decided to sport the wig with a hat I borrowed from Kate. I felt self-conscious all night, but still had a pretty good time. It's weird to go out again. I'm so used to being a homebody and hanging out with my parents. Now that Hilda doesn't have softball, I think I'll be doing more "teenage things." At least I hope. I'm tired of being different. I want to feel young again. My biggest setback is my self-confidence these days. I'm constantly worried about my weight and whether or not it's obvious that I'm bald. Once I'm past this, I have a good time.

Another event that took place last weekend is that on Friday Kate, Lissa, Sandra, and me went to Santa Barbara to see "Live" in concert. This, too, was a big step for me. I stressed for a week about what I was going to wear on my head and body, but in the end we ate pot rice krispie treats and enjoyed the good music and I stressed for no reason.

Yet, on the way back I had a big let down. Kate was telling her sister about a party for Dale she was going to on Saturday. Someone whom I thought was a friend of mine also. She was talking about all the people who would be there and how much fun it would be. I began to feel kinda' uncomfortable. How could someone be so thoughtless to continue to talk about an event she knew I wasn't going to. Her sister then asked me why I wasn't going, and I answered, holding back tears, that it was because I wasn't invited. It was then that Kate replied, "don't look at me... I'm of no authority to invite her." Once again, I felt betrayed. Here is someone I call friend who is claiming that it is out of her control when all she had to do is tell Dale I want to come. Besides, parties don't usually require formal invitations. The real reason behind it was that she was going with Mona and she didn't want to invite me to come with them. So, I've pretty much lost faith in Kate these days. I always thought that Kate didn't invite me to go places because there is nothing to do in this town. Now, I wonder what the true reason is that results in us never doing anything (together). One never knows.

Chapter Fifteen

A day of chemotherapy

Tuesday, May 30, 1995

It's Tuesday and Amber is getting the second part of her fourth cycle of chemo. Red is her favorite nurse, and that name is one of endearment. There are two Ann's working in the office, and this Ann happens to be the one she clicked with. All of the nurses are quite capable and super-sweet but Red feels like family.

Because Amber's chemo has to be administered intravenously, sometimes finding a vein can be a problem. This particular day it is very difficult. Is this going to become a problem in the next few months? There is so much involved in what seems just a routine. First, the nurse has to ascertain which vein appears cooperative. This is an art that only an Oncology Nurse can comprehend.

"Amber, put your hand inside this heating pad for a few minutes. Maybe we can coerce this vein to come out of hiding." Red smiled and went to check on another patient receiving their chemo.

"Mom, could you go get me that People magazine in the lobby. I saw an article on Matt Damon in it." Amber sat patiently with her hand wrapped inside the warm pad. She was wearing her favorite blue and silver paisley silk scarf tied neatly at the nape of her neck, a bow fastidiously fanned out and visible from the front. It was like looking at a model for Vogue. Her make-up just so, her lips colored in the fashionable New York Red, her long eyelashes framing her soft yet striking blue eyes that matched the blue tint of her scarf. She was the youngest in the room, as usual, and she looked out of place seated in the tiny room between two senior citizens.

"Ok, honey." I answered as I got up, sidestepping an I.V. pole with meds hanging down in a clear plastic bag. The room was full. Standing room only. "Do you want something to drink? That might help plump up those veins of yours."

"One of those Crystal Geysers sounds good," she answered quickly, "and maybe a couple of chocolate candies." She added as an afterthought.

I walked to the adjoining building where they kept a refrigerator and a break room for the staff. By now, I had become familiar with the location of any snacks available for the day, including little bowls of assorted candies and even sometimes homemade things brought by other patients for the nurses. They were accustomed to me nosing around during the course of Amber's therapy. Sometimes we were there up to four hours at a time, and it could get pretty boring if I let it. So, I never let it. I was constantly on the move.

"How about anyone else?" I opened to the three other patients in the room. One dozing off, another engrossed in a novel, and the last one taking me up on the offer. I returned with my hands full of goodies to drink, eat, and Amber's magazine.

By this time, Red was ready to check for a possible vein once more.

"Hang your arm down by the chair and keep making a fist, Amber." Red reminded her. "We'll try the usual one."

She flicked the vein with her middle finger, and then proceeded to insert the needle. I knelt down beside Amber on the opposite side, and held her hand.

"Squeeze my hand, honey, and don't look." I focused on my little girl. She was the only person in the room filled with people. There was silence as Red tried fishing around, to no avail.

"I'm sorry, Amber. It is just not cooperating today. I'll have to try on top of your hand." Red apologized with true compassion.

Amber smiled after a wince. "That's ok. I guess I didn't drink enough fluids. I will try to think positive this time, maybe that will help."

Another attempt was made and eventually, victory. The vein held up, and now the therapy could begin.

We carried on our day together as if we were having a simple four-hour visit. People came and went. I helped Amber wheel her I.V. pole into the restroom, and wheel it back to the recliner. When Dr. Dan would stick his nose into the room, we would all say hi, and often he would have some bit of wisdom to impart to Amber, or ask her if she got to watch Seinfeld the night before. It was clear they had a special relationship. She was obviously more than just his patient. They were becoming buddies.

Pulling the needle out was much easier. Amber and I still held hands nevertheless. This was an act that has become a ritual for any pokes she has to have from the weekly blood draws to check her red and white cells and hemoglobin, to the eventual blood transfusions needed when those counts aren't high enough. We will cross that bridge when we come to it. She is doing well so far, no transfusions needed.

Wednesday, June 7, 1995

Amber is feeling a bit better today. Her last "chemo cocktail" made her feel crappy most of the week. Today, I am a little sad thinking of how small her world has become. She depends on me so much, I feel there's nothing left for Bridgett or Tommy. It's like we are on an island and only have each other. I am going to my women's campout this weekend. This will be my first time away since Amber was diagnosed. I'm looking forward to only taking care of my needs. I guess I'm being a little selfish, but I think I need to be for a little while. Maybe I can sort out my feelings for my husband that seem to be non-existent right now. Amber's illness has preoccupied us both, I guess.

First Poke

I hope the needle
won't hurt too much
I say this prayer
with hopes as such

But, prayers are shallow
When dealing with
the unknown evil
the healing myth

My faith is teetering too and fro
I try to grab and not let go
but manage yet
to hold on tight
my mind and body
in tethered flight

Janine

Saturday, June 10, 1995

 Once again I haven't kept up on my journal entries simply because I'm lazy. Life has been plugging along as usual. I'm through with my fourth cycle (chemotherapy) and getting ready to start the fifth on the 26th. Slowly the end is approaching. I can't wait. I'm sick of being fat, bald and tired.

 Sandra is back for the summer, which thrills me. I finally have a friend I can count on. At least I hope so.

 A lot has happened since the last time I wrote. Kurt called and asked what I've been up to. Well, let's see if I can recap the last three and a half months in a brief phone conversation. I had a real hard time being civil to him, but I ended up handling it real well. I don't think we'll be talking again for a while, but I do thing it helped me to come to the realization that I'm better off without him!

 As for the rest of my social life, I took a big step a few weeks back and went to the Graduate nightclub for the first time since I lost my hair. (I didn't enjoy it, but at least I did it.) I put on a wig and a hat and showed up with Hilda. The whole night I was self-conscious about my hair and depressed cause while Hilda was dancing with her boyfriend, I was on the sidelines not getting asked to dance. After that night I decided that the dancing/scamming scene is not for me right now. In fact, that's why I'm home tonight because I refused to go to Tortilla Flats with Hilda and Sandra. They don't understand, but that's because they aren't in my shoes, nor do I think they could handle being there.

Sunday, June 11, 1995

 I am back from the campout and it went by too fast. I stayed busy visiting with friends, attending meetings, hanging out at the beach by the lake, doing exactly nothing but what I wanted to do. The simple freedom of taking care of just myself was very enjoyable. I got to see some women from other parts of the county, including some from last year's campout. My sponsor and dear friend, Marilyn, went with me and we got goofy together when "lights out" came. Our bladders were on the same clock, and we bared it all outside our tent in the dark, wee hours of the morning when Mother Nature called to us. Most of all, we got to talk, talk, really talk, my own needs coming out, along with my fears of controlling Amber too much.

 I also felt some of my spirituality come alive through nature. My connection bonded once again with my Higher Power through the loving exchange of fellow members and friends. I felt renewed.

 God, please help me to keep the feeling of freedom I had at the campout.

Chapter Sixteen

<u>Conflict</u>

Tuesday June 20, 1995

     Spirits couldn't be lower around here. Amber has had a cold, fever and cough for a week. She went to pick up Sandra at UCSB to bring her home for the summer and has been sick ever since. A visit to Dr. Dan and a chest x-ray showed no fluid in her lungs, so that is good. She is so irritable from coughing and feeling sick and that adds to her already low self-esteem because of her physical looks. She has outgrown all her clothes at 132 lbs, and won't go out with her friends because she says people stare at her. She has a thorn up her butt all the time, feeling so different and crying at the drop of a hat. There is nothing I can do for her. She is just a mess.

     I try to cheer her up, but it just doesn't happen for very long. She sees how Sandra is so tan and pretty and her hair is long and beautiful. She feels jealous, then feels bad for being jealous. I keep telling her to have her feelings, but try to pop out of it. This too shall pass; I just need to convince her of that. She feels old, fat, ugly, and unlovable. I need to reassure her that she's beautiful on the inside, outside and lovable. I need the strength to be convincing and to remind myself to let it go and let God work in her life. I can't change what is happening to her, but I can try to present nutritious, non-fattening meals, encourage her to walk with me every day, do Yoga, and keep her brain active by turning off the TV. Things aren't impossible, we just have to jump the hurdles and clear them by being prepared. Spiritually, I feel good and trust that my Higher Power can take up the slack.

Wednesday, June 21, 1995

It's 9:15am, and we've been here at French Hospital since 8:25. Today is Amber's C.A.T. scan to see if the demon is gone from her body. I am confident that no cancer remains and that she is on the road to cure.

She is now in the machine and Lynn is the technician. She is such a sweetie with a smile from ear to ear. This makes it almost bearable. Ok, now Dr. Kim has her I.V. in, the iodine will go through her veins and help complete the pictures needed for the scan. That, combined with the Redi-cat she drank last night and this morning, will light up her body and show her vital organs. Now, the recording of Lynn's voice to "take a deep breath…" repeated over and over again as her body inches through the huge tunnel of the x-ray machine.

As I sit right next door, I feel closer to her and can almost pretend it's happening to me. Its almost 10:00 and she's been breathing and holding for about seven minutes. The last time we were here was like a bad dream. This time we know what to expect and there is a feeling of accomplishment knowing the results will show a reduction in the size of the mass in her sternum. After all, she has been going through chemotherapy for four months. There has to be a change for the better. I know she still has two more cycles of chemo to go, and her resistance to infection is waning. I just know for today she is feeling better with her cold and cough and she slept better last night. These are little victories now, leading up to the big one.

Wednesday, June 21, 1995

If I had one wish in the world, it would be that this hell that I'm living would all be just a really bad dream. I'm sick of it! I'm tired of being different then every teen my age. I went out with Sandra tonight and saw "Batman Forever." We had a really good time, but then two of her friends from UCSB came to visit. Let's just say I hate meeting Sandra's friends who have heard so much about me and seen pictures and then they see me in person and they look at me with this pathetic look like, "it sucks to be you." Yeah, well, I know it sucks to be me. This introduction was no different. We went to Sandra's house and there was Hilda with two of her friends. Once again, I'm introduced and everyone's uncomfortable because I'm fat and wearing a scarf to cover up my baldhead. Even Hilda was acting weird.

Eventually, me, Sandra and her two friends went to her bedroom. They began talking about UCSB and then the Lake Havasu excursion and immediately I feel like someone on the outside looking in. I have no stories to tell nor do they care. I felt like a reject. Then one of the girls starts looking through old pictures of me and Sandra and asks her "Who the pretty blond is." Yeah, well it used to be me. I felt humiliated. She tried to cover up by saying "Every one looks different," but I was the only one in the pictures. I felt like saying, "Thanks for pointing out that I turned ugly with chemotherapy."

The next letdown, Hilda walked in and started talking about going to the lake this weekend, which I've never heard anything about, so apparently I'm not included. (Not saying I would go, but it just seemed like I was being constantly reminded of how much my life has changed.)

Finally, I couldn't take anymore and as I was leaving one of the girls asked if I would be joining them tomorrow at the beach. Yeah right. Like I really want to lay out with a bunch of skinny, longhaired, pretty girls at the beach. I would stick out like a sore thumb, not to mention get laughed at. I would give anything to look like I used to last summer. I used to be Sandra's beach buddy, now she goes with Hilda. I used to be her Graduate buddy, too. Now she goes with Hilda.

It really sucks. Not only do I have to have a disease and go through the temporary changes of losing hair and gaining weight, but also I can't do the fun things everyone else does and get my mind off of it. I'm constantly reminded that I'm different and ALONE.

ALONE is where I'll be tomorrow while all of those girls are catching rays and scammin' on guys at Avila Beach.

ALONE is how I'll feel each and everyday until this nightmare ends.

Chapter Nineteen

Good News, Bad News

Saturday, June 24, 1995

     It is a sunny day and everyone is still asleep. The birds are chirping and it is so quiet. Today I feel better. Yesterday I was a little down and depressed. Tom and I went to our Marriage Encounter group meeting and we talked about our early dating days and the romance and love that goes with the courting process. I laughed when we reminisced about drive-in movies, watching TV late at night together, making out on the couch. Everyone shared his or her experiences. It was fun.

     While we were gone, Amber and Bridgett went to Sandra's house and soaked in the hot tub and watched a movie. Amber was looking forward to the evening and was in a great mood. I love it when her sister takes her out and spends time with her. It is good for both of them. So little of our previous lives' activities are intact. The disease monopolizes every waking moment. Chemotherapy treatments and the effects from them fill our days. Worry about the next scan fills our nights.

     Today Amber will go to Santa Margarita to be with some friends from college. I hope it goes OK. She has been so unhappy with her body and doesn't want to go anywhere. Some of these friends haven't seen her since the whole ordeal began. Now without hair and 20 lbs heavier, her self-esteem is fragile to say the least.

But, today is a good day right now and I'm going to enjoy myself one moment at a time. I am powerless over Amber's friends and whether they accept her or not. I can only catch her when she falls, I cannot prevent her from tumbling.

Monday, June 26, 1995

Our appointment with Dr. Dan today will tell the story of the latest scan. Now it's time to show her pictures. The good doc puts them up for us to see. The blackened, grayish areas against the white of the bone structure consistently confuse me. (Once I saw this huge thing on the side of her lung, I gasped; it was her heart.) The science of reading x-rays definitely takes they eye of a qualified physician to read.

Standing there, staring at the inside of her body, feels like barging in on something very private. Discussing her inner body parts, flipping through x-ray after x-ray, the trained eye of Dr. Dan makes sense of it all. I listen for voice intonation and watch for positive body language and facial expression. Amber watches intently, my gaze goes between her reaction and his. He is her lifeline, the teller of her fate. How fragile is the balance between ease and disease. He points to the mass in question, next to the sternum. Amazingly there is a 99.9% decrease in disease size. This is great news to me, but does not warrant the end of chemotherapy treatments. After number six there will be another scan. If the tumor continues to decrease in size then more chemo will be necessary, but if the size stays the same then it is scar tissue and no more chemo is needed. Weird. It seems like it should be the other way around. It's not like a big eraser that goes in and deletes the disease completely. After killing the beast with poison, the carcass still remains unchanged in size. Therefore, if it keeps getting smaller there is a pinpoint of a cancer cell present that needs to be attacked until it lies motionless; helpless in a sea of poisonous drugs unable to rear it's ugly head. Period. End of story. We pray for this type of ending. A happy one where all the evil, black cancer cells are eradicated and the good white ones win.

Once the pictures are discussed, treatment number five gets underway. The first I.V. didn't reach a vein, so a second poke is done. Bingo. I hate to see her have to get stuck twice. Her veins are building up scar tissue. It's as if they know the needle is coming and shift mysteriously in avoidance.

I sit next to my little girl holding her free hand for the poke. Now we will settle in for the drip of the anti-emetic that will help prevent nausea from the drugs she will receive shortly afterward. Once the I.V. is in I feel relief. The entire process will take the remainder of the day. I would rather be here with Amber than anywhere else in the world.

Chemotherapy 101

I looked around and I saw

empty eyes

>   staring at the wall

The evidence of one

>   too young to sit there

Waiting for the meds

>   the poke——somewhere…

I see the end

>   This road's too long

 I see myself

>   as one who helps, but not enough

My hands are tied

>   I'm against the wall

I want to scream

>   don't fall… don't fall

Just take your time

>   it won't take long

Some thirty years

>   squeezed into

One.

Janine

Chapter Twenty

<u>Life on life's terms</u>

June 30, 1995

    I got back my C/T scans on Monday and began my 5th cycle. The news for the most part was good. Everything had decreased and all that remains is a 3cm x 4cm mass behind my sternum. I thought this would be the day I would find out about when my last cycle would be, but until we have two consecutive x-rays that show the mass is merely residual, he can't commit to only six cycles. Therefore, I [won't] find out if six is the last until after [treatment] six when I get another C/T scan. Despite the uncertainty I'm trying to keep thinking positive and am imagining myself done after the sixth.

    Tomorrow me and the fam are scheduled to go "canoeing" with Dr. Dan and his wife, "Ped's Patti and her family and a few others we met from camp Reach for the Star's.

    I'm thankful that I got to know my doctor on a different level because he's more than just the cancer specialist he's my friend. Same goes for the nurses I've got to know well. Like Patti and Debbie. I can really say I've got the chance to meet some really special people through this all, friends whom I hope to keep forever.

Thursday, July 6, 1995

The sun is out—-yes. It feels like the calm before the storm. I am alone. Amber is outside sitting in the sun and Bridgett is at school, Tom at work. I hear the wind chimes playing their song and the chirping birds singing along. Faintly I hear the surf landing on the beach and see it from my dining room window. Who needs to go away on vacation when it's right here?

I've been feeling sorry for myself that we can't afford to go some place special to celebrate Amber's last cycle of chemo. In fact, we don't even know if it will be her last one. The next C.A.T. scan will tell. Sometimes I get so sad and worried about Amber. She is getting weaker and weaker. She can't turn on the shower handle with one hand nor shuffle cards with both. When squatting down to pick up something, she has trouble getting back up. The stairs to the back yard are a chore and there are only four of them. This is hardly the physical strength of a typical 19 year old.

I can see the frustration on her face, but she snaps out of it quickly, afraid to let any one down, or to worry me. Trying so desperately to be like others her age. At least Sandra spent some time over here with her yesterday. That helped a lot. I feel so helpless.

Monday, July 10, 1995

I'm sitting here listening to the joyful sound of the vacuum cleaner. Bridgett is doing her chores. It's 10:00 am and she's getting them done early (at my request) before anything else. It looks like it may be another rocky week aboard this ship. Her teenage hormones are flaring up and having a civil conversation is impossible. The best offence for her is defense. As parents we try to include her in our activities. We know she has been slighted during this family ordeal, but there is no pleasing her.

With her sister gone to Yosemite for her annual trip with Sandra's family, we thought we might patch up our differences, but she is a foreigner in our home. Taking her to a movie was like forcing her to go to a funeral. Of course the preference was to go with her friends. Beware of expectations. They are pre-meditated resentments. And how. I am trying very hard to remember that she is individuating and this is typical of a teen development thing.

Meanwhile, I am trying to get excited about my own life change. The orientation for Cal Poly in San Luis Obispo was yesterday. I have planned out my tentative schedule and am taking twelve units. This will be a real challenge to stay focused on college classes while my sweet baby is going through chemo. I don't know if I can pull it off.

Amber called and sounds good even though she is not able to do the things she has been accustomed to. Last year she and Sandra hiked up to the top of Half Dome. Even experienced hikers have trouble doing that. I'm so grateful she got to reach such a pinnacle in her life before she got sick. The strength and stamina it took to accomplish that is nothing compared to the courage it is taking to get through the ordeal of having cancer.

Having her gone is hard. I miss her. We have become very close. I've been thinking a lot about whether this is her last cycle of chemo. God's will is the way it must be. I must keep the faith.

Monday, July 17, 1995

Finally Bridgett is coming around. She has blossomed since her sister has been gone. I took her shopping yesterday and she was quite appreciative. Thanking me over and over, I enjoyed every minute of our time together. Later in the evening Tom and I took her bowling and had a blast. I want to pay more attention to her and keep this in mind when Amber comes home.

Chapter Twenty-one

<u>Beware of Hidden Agendas</u>

Tuesday, July 18, 1995

The sun is shining somewhere, just not here. Inside my heart is gloomy as well. Bridgett has been like a different child, in a good way, while Amber was gone, but the weekend before she was to come back home, all hell broke loose. Not only was she busted for spending the night at a friend's house without adult supervision, (a confession she made the day after) there was a bigger problem ahead.

Honest, I wasn't snooping, although I am not beyond reproach and have been known to read a page or two of her so-called hidden journal when desperate for an explanation of her foul moods. As I was putting something back on her closet shelf something was in the way. I had to reach deeply to retrieve a small wallet. As I looked through the change part there was something crumpled up. I sought out some good lighting and looked at it more closely.

It was green. I touched it, smelled it. I was in big denial here. It couldn't be. It had to be bark from a tree, or something. I put it down, walked to my room, and walked back, more like a frantic sort of pacing. Finally, I decided to light it up and smell it. I wasn't a teenager of the sixties for nothing. Bingo. The acrid, unmistakable smell of pot filled my nose. Oh my God, she had a stash of pot.

So much went through my head. How could this be? I decided to wait until

Tom got home from work. She was supposed to tell her Dad about her first offence. He would be very surprised about this one.

We sat down to discuss the problem of her lying to us about spending the night. That was when I went to get the wallet and set it on the table in front of her.

"Where did you get that?" Bridgett was sweating bullets. She looked at me wide-eyed and puzzled.

"In your closet hidden on a shelf. Can you explain?" I wasn't letting her off easy and neither was her father.

She began by saying she hadn't tried pot in a long time. Which means? This was not the first time. Oh, shit.

We were at the part about consequences for her actions, and had received her "I'm sorry Mom and Dad," hugs and promises to talk more later when the Stribling family pulled into the driveway. Amber was home from her trip. What a homecoming, I thought. Now she would have to witness the hard part. Sentencing.

"Grounded for ten days? And I can't spend the night with anyone for a whole month? How could you? That's not fair." The tears are abundant and quickly become bitter. "I hope you know my summer is ruined."

Mine, too, I thought. Enforcing punishment is no easy task, but least we didn't outlaw television. Having learned something over the years, we discovered that particular punishment was harder on the punisher (parents) than the punishee (child.) These teenage years counted for double trouble.

The evening went on, Amber filling us in with her trip news, which wasn't good. She was bummed a lot of the time due to her lack of energy. How do you go back to a place like Yosemite with its memories of hiking Half Dome and scamming on guys? This was certainly difficult for her to realize and accept the weight gain, hair loss, the tone of the entire trip was changed from previous years.

We had gone from one battle zone into another. Bridgett was locked in her room, and Amber was down in the dumps headed to hers. Wasn't it the mother's job to keep her children safe, healthy, and happy? I was beginning to let the whole thing get to me. Feeling like a failure, I sat down and wept.

Tuesday, August 6, 1995

Wow it's been a while. Things are going ok around here. Actually not ok. My parents always fight about something. I'm always in trouble and my sister sits on her high pedestal and cries. I know I'm stupid. Ok my sister has cancer and I'm thinking of myself. These feelings have to be normal. I don't know. Anyway what I really wanted to write about is <u>my</u> life for once. You're probably the only one who really cares right now. Yes I am feeling sorry for myself. This is normal too! (right?) Am I retarded?

BC

Chapter Twenty-two

<u>New Friends</u>

Monday, August 7, 1995

    A real coincidence happened today. While we were waiting for Amber's treatment number six, we met a family that my friend Karen is acquainted with. She mentioned that their 17 year old daughter, Erin, had been diagnosed with cancer recently and she wanted us to meet them. As it turned out, she is also one of Dr. Dan's patients. Her parents and I sat and talked in the lobby of the doctor's office as our girls received their treatments at the same time. They shared their experience and how this disease had changed their lives and how the friends have dwindled and blown away for their daughter. They seem to be ok, but one never knows. I seem ok on the surface most of the time, too. This is serious stuff any way you put it. I'm really glad we finally got to meet. This is in God's time. We have to be silent sometimes and really listen and wait. Meeting them like this is quite fortunate, as we probably would have never met otherwise. Between hospital procedures, staging of the cancer, illness due to chemotherapy, the possibility of scheduling a meeting was almost nil. For some reason it is comforting to meet another family going through this hell. Sharing the ups and downs is therapeutic. Erin has two siblings, an older brother and younger sister. As in our case, the diagnosis was a complete shock.

    Erin has a very rare type of cancer called PNET. It essentially is a tumor that usually forms on the brain, but hers developed on her neck at about the same spot as Amber did. Her chemotherapy treatments will be far more aggressive as the tumor for this type of cancer tends to grow quickly. She is a junior at the same high school Amber attended. They shared the stories of hair loss and friend loss, and actually were able to laugh about it.

   We have exchanged phone numbers and have vowed to get together as two families fighting similar battles. It is an odd thing to have in common, but more importantly we are possible ports for each other in the many storms to come.

Erin's War

A battle waged
she's many years beyond her age
Her body cries
enough already!
Counts rise and fall
fight to be steady
Such spirit I
shall never see
Just feisty, strong
not grim for she
has brushed with death
victoriously
and shone true grit
gloriously
Hang on tight
the battles' building
Stay staunch and strong
remain unflinching
Fight tooth and nail
reach down inside
Pull out defenses that want to hide
Reach way down deep
the strength is there
Refuse to quit and show
NO FEAR!!!

Chapter Twenty-three

<u>Birthdays Should Be Happy</u>

August 8, 1995

 Well, it's my birthday and once again I'm reminded of all that used to be. I haven't written in my journal lately because I feel as though it hurts more to repeat what I've been through each day. I've had some tough weeks or should I say a couple of months. In brief, I went to Tahoe and Yosemite in July and returned depressed because I'm still different. Luckily, my hair has started to grow back and I didn't have to wear a scarf, but people still stared (at me) the same. Boys didn't look at me…only Sandra, and after nine days, I came home and exploded. I pretty much stayed this sad for the month of July.

 Upon my return my friendship with Sandra has seemed to drift away. She has chosen to continue her life in the social scene without me. She goes to the Grad night club, hangs out with old friends, parties at Santa Barbara and I get the privilege of hearing about all of it detail for detail which drives me crazy. I DON'T CARE! She doesn't realize that it makes things worse when I'm constantly reminded what I'm missing out on. I find that presently I have nothing in common with her. So I (have) started to avoid her.

 Another let down that topped off my mood was the postponement of treatment number six because of a low WBC. [white blood count] This threw everything a week off which meant treatment ABV [adriamycin, bleomycin, vincristine] would be given to me the day before my birthday. Plus, it would be longer before I would find out whether or not this is my last. So basically it bummed me out. Nothing felt like it was working out.

It was then that I was invited to Santa Barbara by Abby for Fiesta. I "thought" it would be a good idea to get away for an evening and hopefully have some fun. Little did I know that this, too, would be a disaster.

The day went fine, but mine and Abby's idea for the night were completely opposite. She wanted to drink and go to a party. I obviously didn't because I couldn't. I told her exactly how I felt about parties and thought she got the point, but despite my feelings she got drunk by herself and we ended up at a party. Nervous to walk in, I attempted to put my fears aside and try to be strong. After all I wasn't going to know anyone, I wasn't going to drink and I knew people were going to look at me funny. No sooner were we at the gate when my worst night-mare came true. The guy charging for the keg called me a guy in front of everyone then started laughing when he realized his mistake. I immediately started crying and wanted to leave, but Abby wasn't as cooperative especially because she had been drinking. This was (the) worst I had felt in a long time. Some people can be so rude and insensitive! And people wonder why I don't go out. If they only knew how hard it is to maintain self worth going through what I have in today's society. They would not be able to handle it.

Tuesday, August 8, 1995

This year Amber's birthday is something to be extra grateful for. Even though it is not the happiest of times, still it remains to be cause to celebrate her life. When all else fails to bring me out of the depths of depression, I can reminisce about the actual day of her birth.

At 4:30 a.m. a beautiful pink baby girl weighing 6 lbs 12 oz slid out after only a few hours of labor. My recollection of that moment is very clear, when her father held up the hand mirror so I could see her come into the world. He was allowed be in the delivery room with me to be my coach and see the miracle of birth. Our first-born daughter entered the world without any drugs in my body so she was alert and curious from the beginning.

All ten fingers and toes, and a bushel of light brown hair crowning her head, her daddy whisked her off to the nursery. As he proudly carried the tiny bundle, she chris-tened him with her first present, and a wet blanket for proof. It was a story he would tell many times, much to Amber's dismay, and usually to an unsuspecting boyfriend.

Indeed, there are few moments that please me more to remember. It was the first of many that would come straight from my heart.

We have sure been through a rough time in the present. She has weathered the storm and I like to think I have helped her do that. And she has helped me. Sometimes I just feel like I failed somehow, somewhere to keep this terrible thing from happening to her. I should be able to protect her from all harm. I know how Mary must have felt when Jesus was on the cross, watching his pain and anguish and fighting the fear gripping her.

BEING A CHILD

Looking back at long ago
I began to miss the innocence I once possessed.
As a small child, I had no worries in the world.
My biggest concern
Was what toy I was going to play with that day

I want so much to be
That child again
And rid myself
Of the realities of life.
To run away from
The coldness of the world
And be happy every waking minute.

It is these times
When, by myself
Thinking about my troubles,
That I wish
I could be a child again.

Amber Carter

Chapter Twenty-four

Guests or Pests?

Wednesday, August 16, 1995

Having company, even grandparents all the way from Albuquerque, was not easy. Our lives had been a series of updates to them through long distance phone calls for the last six months. A thousand miles is a big buffer for bad news. No one in my extended family aside from mom had ventured into our world, much less friends we had here. We wanted it that way. I guess it was just easier.

When it came time to entertain them, I was not up to it. We were up to our eyeballs with chemotherapy, CBC's, C.T. scans, special diets, hair loss, mood swings and an occasional breakdown or two. This is the world of a family with cancer. Yes, the entire family has it in one form or another. As captain of denial, it was my job to be cheerleader, spokeswoman, and all around firewatcher. I could make dinner, give Amber her neupogen shot, juggle an argument between Tom and Bridgett, and pay the bills while I studied for finals. No problem. But add Grandpa to the picture and I felt like having a Valium cocktail. By day five, I was certifiably ready for the local nut farm. Luckily they left for Yuma in the nick of time, apologizing for their short stay. The family was ecstatic.

Don't get me wrong. They meant well. It's just that our family mobile was barely balancing as it was. Adding two more made it really go out of whack quickly. If I had any advice to give to people about visiting a family in crisis, I would suggest NOT doing it. Send money instead.

Now, having my mother here in March was just the ticket at the time. She helped us deal with the early diagnosis by doing the laundry, cooking dinners, making Amber's special herbal tea that boost her immune system and simply being quietly helpful. She was not just a visitor; she was part of our unit. She helped immeasurably. So I correct my previous statement. Send money and my mother.

Chapter Twenty-five

College of hard knocks

Monday, August 21, 1995

Amber is off to school, her first day at Hancock Community College. This will be an interim move towards her goal of transferring back to USD after this ordeal is over.

I pray that she has a positive experience today and that she comes home brimming with good news and a positive attitude. This is where she needs to be. School has always been her element. It will give her purpose and some unique experiences to share with her last remaining friend, Sandra. Amazing how all others have forsaken her. In all fairness to her friends, Amber has played a part in that by isolating herself also, but she learned to do that out of self-preservation. It hurts her too much to be rejected.

Thursday, August 24, 1995

This has been hell week. Monday: "I don't have anyone to eat lunch with and I have a two hour break today." Tears fall from her sweet round face. I go into my pep talk mode, become her best cheerleader and reiterate what I've told her 1000 times before—"You are special, smart, pretty, loyal and caring. You'll meet people in smaller groups that will recognize that in you." Tuesday: "OK, so the Geology class is fun—the lab offers you a chance to meet Jess, a cute guy who is in your group, that's great! See, I told you so." Inside this mom is overflowing with gratitude that my prayers were answered. Finally, I see a parting of the dark cloud cover that hovers over her head these days. Good thing I had been able to find some time to talk to friends in the program and vent my feelings this morning. Thank you Sue, Ann, and Donna. You all listened while I let it go.

Chapter Twenty-six

<u>Take a deep breath, hold it, breathe...</u>

Friday, August 25, 1995

Let me begin by saying that we do not know how fragile we are, nor do we fully understand how incredibly strong we can be. When I think of the amount of time Amber has spent inside a machine while her body is being x-rayed, I am reminded how patient, brave and willing she is to do whatever is asked of her. If you include hours of chemotherapy, doctor's appointments, weekly blood draws, and all the waiting involved and dependence on health care workers to do their job, there is an amazing amount of trust, patience, and courage required. She is anything but fragile.

Weekly stabs to her veins are needed to test her precious blood. For every cancer cell that is eradicated a white cell meets the same fate. The results are blood transfusions intended to add new white and red ones to fight the battle. When the platelets suffer losses, those are replaced as well. When they are low there is a real danger of the blood's inability to clot, making it a dangerous situation in the case of an injury. Even having a menstrual period or a razor cut from shaving her legs could mean a possible hemorrhage. As if this is not enough to keep her on the edge of insanity, there are regular C.A.T. scans done, and x-rays that reveal what is or is not still there trying to kill her.

But to the average eye, she is just regular type person with a slightly irregular hair-do, sort of like a pixie without the pointed ears. She keeps the smile she was born with on her porcelain face. Not only is her skin pure, so is her soul. She is impeccable about her make-up and clothes. Even if she is only sitting in a chair for six hours receiving chemotherapy, that scarf on her head better match her outfit.

So, this is what I do while I am waiting. I write. Countless hours spent traveling to the hospitals, labs, and imaging centers, sitting in waiting rooms with outdated magazines lying on the end tables, people watching. No wonder soap operas are filmed in make-believe hospitals. There is so much not to do here. I carry her own blanket and pillow with us when she receives blood products. It brings some warm fuzzies from home. From now on, home is where we are. Have afghan, will travel.

Her time for the scan is drawing to a close. I can hear Lynne from my perch in the dressing room next to the scanner. "Take a deep breath…hold it…breathe." Click. Then over and over until her voice lulls me into a stupor. Silence. It is over. Now to wait for results. More waiting.

At this point in time I am having two completely incompatible thoughts. One, her disease is gone and she's cured and the bells ring, confetti flies, there are smiles and laughter and a sense of relief pours over me.

The other is a grim picture of the mundane task of more chemotherapy, how much who knows, more visits to Dr. Dan, bloating of Amber's face and body, tears and many more feelings that I can't write down here and now.

I must not give into despair. I have to be strong and positive for her sake. She is feeling it times one hundred and she's still putting one foot in front of the other and so can I. This Sunday there will be a mass said for her and the prayers of our church community will give her hope. I need to hold onto that hope right now. It's all I have.

Interlude

Amber's hair had been curled in the pink sponge rollers overnight. With care and pride I parted it down the center and made two ponytails that held the tiniest of shiny curls on either side of her head.

The black leotard and pink tights were slightly baggy as she was a tiny little thing. Posed in the kitchen with her pink ballet shoes on, her smile of sheer delight warmed my heart.

Here was my first-born daughter, pink and pretty, shining like a new penny. Eager to dance and accustomed to the teacher and dance studio, she hadn't a worry in the world. Miss Winnie would be gentle and loving and trustworthy.

I took a picture of my little ballerina as she pointed her toe out to the side. Click—a moment caught in time. Motherhood was never better. Here I was, getting ready to whisk my three-year old baby girl off to her first dance class where she would do ballet, tap, and tumbling.

Raised in the studio atmosphere from conception, it was a most natural order of things for her. When she turned three there would be the beginning of formal dance class, but she knew it already. Hadn't those little feet covered every inch of the dance floor the past two years? From the time she was able to hold on to her walker on wheels and push from her toes and cruise around, she was a natural. Amber was constantly with me as I taught dance and took my own classes. She was in her comfort zone.

Was I ready to let her go? I thought so. There would be many firsts for my little dancer, but she was always ready and willing to start new things. No tears or clinging to Mommy. Oh, no. When the time came she was off and ready with not even a look back.

Eager to please and innocent of haste, she and only one other child took their first class together. I thank God for that beginning, an extension of myself standing there in first position ready to conquer the world, then skip happily back to Mommy's lap to grin and share the new experience.

Chapter Twenty-seven

Loss of sacred trust

Thursday, August 31, 1995

This month is gone and it is not leaving with a whimper. After six long months of treatments, the tumor behind Amber's sternum is still shrinking. The cancer still lurks insidiously. As a sort of ritual, and in support of Amber, our family always went with her to have the C.A.T. scans read. Dr. Dan made it a point to place the x-rays up for us all to see. He would then explain them in detail and answer any questions.

Typically, he was neutral before the viewing. Careful not to divulge any hint of pending results, he would blandly say hello without emotion and proceed to the inner sanctum where systematically, in due time they became known through his painstaking procedure.

This day he was visibly different, jovial and even asking Amber if she "felt lucky" today. We were all lulled into a perky, positive atmosphere. But that soon became a cruel façade. The results were anything but favorable as he placed the pictures up and began reading them. I can only figure that he hadn't had time to actually pre-read the x-rays and therefore was talking out of his ass, so to speak.

When Amber began to cry, he tried to console her, but of course, that was impossible. She had been duped into believing there was good news to share when the facts were quite the opposite. No cajoling on his part would take away the disappointment she felt, we all felt. If I could have moved, I would have slapped him in the face. As it was, I was so shocked, I was motionless and speechless as was our entire family.

Eventually the appointment ended, but not the pain of the previous indiscretion. We were herded out the door with our hearts in our hands and the feeling of starting over from square one. I had an ache in my heart and a lump in my throat. All I could do was walk away before I said something I would regret. Always afraid I would turn the doctor against her through my condemnation, questions, doubts, I had held my tongue so many times. But this time I would not.

No matter what had happened the previous day, Amber still woke up with a smile on her face. "I love you, Mom," the image I'll never forget—through it all she could still wake up smiling. God gave us strength to help her get through this one day at a time. On this next day Amber's acceptance came quickly. She grieved and cried a lot and got her feelings out. This had been playing on her mind the entire weekend before her appointment.

So I put a Band-Aid on Amber's wounded heart and went along with the doctor. A sleepless night thinking about how he presented her results to us left me pissed off. I couldn't let go of it. Finally she also expressed to me the mixed message she had also gotten from his presentation. Feeling confident of a cheery outcome, lulled into the possibility of an unchanged scan because of his jovial manner, then the elevator came crashing down with the words, "And I think you need two more, don't you?"

His act was over. He was now the bad guy and I want to scratch his eyes out. Instead, I just stroked Amber's back, trying to feel like an adult who needs to hold it all together. How could we let the charade go on and on while she hung on his every word, and then had to watch her break down and crumble before our eyes? Bridgett was big-eyed, but mostly oblivious of the importance of the judgment call, and just glad "My sister is alive," not so much concerned with her quality of life, just that it's there at all. She is a realist.

As we got home, Tom was saying how God had let him down, and why bother to pray or do a mass for her when nothing works. He was mad. So mad and disappointed that he had placed his faith, what was left of it, in God's hands and He just opened his fingers and let us slide on through. We went down to the beach and I tried to talk to him and defend God to no avail. I have learned that we each handle this differently. I haven't lost my faith in God; He's the one holding us together. There is a random evil out there that makes these things happen.

On Friday morning I called Dr. Dan's office to see if I could meet with him, alone. He was going to get a piece of what was left of my mind. Instead I was connected with Red, our favorite nurse. I explained emphatically what had transpired at our last meeting. She assured me that the doctor certainly had not meant any harm. I really wanted to verbally punch his lights out and was pumped up enough to do so no matter what the consequences. She continued to stick up for him and finally agreed to talk to him herself on our behalf if that was all right with me. It was better than nothing, and since I was getting nowhere, I backed down. Don't mess with a mother bear; believe me, we are dangerous. I have to admit that I couldn't have envisioned a better outcome if I had planned it myself.

As we sat in the lobby that following afternoon, Dr. Dan came in and sat down, looking Amber straight in the eye. He proceeded to apologize for the way he handled the previous visit. I was in awe as Amber graciously accepted, yet didn't minimize her feelings by saying, "That's ok". Amber never knew about my phone call and I don't have any way of knowing if he would have done this without it. All I cared about was that Amber continued to have complete faith in this man to go on. She needed to know he was on her side, and also to be able to admit he was wrong. He had been shrunk down in her eyes and this brought him back up to life size where he belonged. Not as God, nor even God-like, just an intelligent, informed specialist in his field. More importantly, one with a heart and some humility.

We went on with the afternoon chemo treatment as usual, but I had a new respect for the human side of this special man. Amber gained respect for herself in that she deserved that apology, and faith that he is her advocate in this union of patient and doctor. We affirmed our one goal in common, to cure her of this terrible disease, and leave her with the respect and dignity she deserves.

Bridgett Speaks Out

Thursday, September 7, 1995

    I am now going into my junior year. Just got my license which is cool but I don't ever get to drive. I really feel like that ever since my sister got sick that my Mom has no idea what is happening in my life. I am really growing up. All these things that I'm going through, getting my license, turning <u>16</u>, getting screwed over by guys, sex, drugs. She has no clue how important this time of my life is for me. My friend Tara has the best relationship with her mom. I want that so bad. Before my Mom knows it I'm going to be out of the house and in college. She's going to wonder how I grew up so fast. It makes me very upset to think I have nobody to share these experiences with. I just want my Mom back!

    BC

Chapter Twenty-eight

<u>Sweet smell of success</u>

Wednesday, September 13, 1995

Yesterday's happiness made up for a lot of sadness in our house. We surprised Bridgett with a belated sixteenth birthday present. Her reaction and look of total surprise when she saw it in the driveway was worth the investment in the 1964 Plymouth two-door. For a whole $400 we made her the happiest teenager on earth. It made us all happy. She finally feels special and deserves the freedom having her own car will give her. It has been a tough six months for her being in the shadow of her sister as she received all the attention. Knowing this must be hard for her to accept. After all, she loves her "sissy" with all her heart and must have trouble understanding the resentment she must feel for the lack of effort on our part. Surely there has been no other way. If there were such a thing, I would have gladly given anything for it. For today we found the magic pill. Let us rejoice.

Along with that surprise, I have been cooking up an "Amber's Angels" club with members from a long list of close friends and relatives. I challenged everyone we know to send Amber a card or letter of encouragement and TLC to lift her spirits after the let down of continued chemotherapy. The response has been incredible. She is receiving mail every day. She smiles and I know she's happy. We all could use plenty of that right now.

With Dr. Dan's ok, Amber started Weight Watchers and I am tagging along for support. Of course losing weight could only benefit us both. It is also a special time we can be together at meetings and receive positive ideas to keep us motivated to lose pounds and with success increase the self-esteem she has been lacking big time.

I relish in the vision of her sitting there, listening to speakers that build self-esteem and encouragement for taking positive action. Improving self-acceptance and being there to witness the transformation of my child to an adult taking hold of her destiny. This is a proactive approach that I hope will carry over to the biggest secret obstacle she faces. Cancer. Also known as the big elephant that sits in our living room and everyone walks around it as if it is not there. Once in awhile it lifts it's ugly trunk up and snorts loudly and becomes obnoxious, but we have all learned to ignore it and get on with the business of living.

When dread and sadness creep back in, we shovel it out like poop from the elephant and hide it in the backyard to use for fertilizer. What else would a family do? Don't we all have some poop to shovel out once in awhile? Ours just seems to multiply. We must quit feeding it so much.

Chapter Twenty-nine

Abnormal is normal

Thursday, September 14, 1995

That didn't last long. The happiness. Once again time to shovel. It's gaining on me. Is my life full of it for some unknown reason? Just how much stress can a parent take?

Bridgett was allowed to take her car out for the first time. The plan was to pick up three girlfriends and go bowling down in Pismo Beach. Now I know boys are usually in the picture, but that's common at this age. What is not common is to get a call from the sheriff's department to go and pick up your daughter. She was being detained by officers for reckless driving in a residential area.

My heart was in my throat and I was shaking and also mad as hell. Her father was calm and cool. His younger days offered the first hand experience necessary to handle a situation of this type. When we pulled up to the street where they were holding her, three boys were propped up on the trunk of her car, surrounded by two police cars. My stomach turned. Lots of questions ran through my mind. Like, where are the girls, and who are these boys, and what happened to the bowling alley?

As we approach, Bridgett comes running towards us. The plain clothes officer tells her to stay put and he proceeds to talk to us privately. Apparently she was speeding around the corner, tires squealing, and there was a party going on at a house nearby (where her girlfriends were.) Answer to at least one of my questions. A neighbor complained about the noise and no parental supervision. Bingo.

The one break we received was that of the officer didn't issue her a ticket or impound the car. He figured that would only fall on our shoulders as punishment through higher insurance rates. Thank you. Now what do we do with this teen who used to be our sweet little daughter?

Of course her side of the story was quite different, as it always is. On the way home she told me how her intention was just to show the boys her car and then go bowling. Right. What about the girlfriends stuck at the party? I guess they walked home. Bridgett cried and cried. She knew this meant no car for a while. She had a taste of freedom and what a bad decision can do. I see it as a test for us—just what we need, another test—shit. I'm damn tired of being tested. I now have a few more gray hairs. The call from the sheriff's department at 9:30pm was a terrifying experience. Calls like that can mean life or death. Hadn't we dealt with the possibility of the latter enough? And so, where do we go from here? Bed, and pull the covers over our heads. Period.

Chapter Thirty

<u>No guarantees</u>

Saturday, September 23, 1995

What a week this was. I am in college and overwhelmed. What was I thinking? Can I keep up this pace? Who will care for Amber while I'm away at school? I know these plans were made long ago, but can I still do it?

Amber is sick right now with a fever and has been home all week, not able to go to her own college classes. Leaving her alone is making me feel guilty. The guilt hammer is pounding me over the head. She had to go for her CBC alone this week. It's the first time I wasn't there to hold her hand while they took her blood. She says not to worry, but that's not possible. Telephone calls from campus help, and I know she needs to be on her own sometimes.

It is such a privilege for me to attend college at my age, and I am grateful every day for this opportunity. I just wish the timing was better. I am a mom first, a student last. The good news is that the rest of the family is taking on responsibilities in my absence. Laundry, cooking, cleaning is being done by someone other than me.

Friday, September 29, 1995

This is the end of my third week in school and I'm feeling better about being there. Tests are looming around the corner, but I'm keeping up with my reading.

Amber is happy today. Her chemo was postponed due to low blood counts. Sandra is in town and tonight they are going to a movie together. I love to see her having fun with her friend. She needs someone young to talk to and share feelings with.

She was noticing her hair loss, evidence on her pillow when she wakes up in the morning. Sometimes I rush in there when she's using the bathroom and brush it off before she can put her glasses on. She is like an eagle swooping to collect it for a nest, noticing every single hair. Yes, I fear the same thing. That she will be bald again and forced to wear the wig, or scarves or just not go out at all. I would give anything to spare her that pain.

"Amber's Angels" are filling the mailbox every day. We are truly blessed for their sincerity. I'm glad I started her club. At least I can feel like I'm doing something constructive and hopeful, knowing I have some control over at least a part of Amber's psyche recovery. She deserves so much more, but at least this makes her smile.

Sunday, October 1, 1995

It's a sunny day, the breeze is blowing off the ocean and I'm determined to get my reading done so we can go down to the beach today. I just talked to my mom as our usual Sunday ritual and it's almost like having her here. She is such a positive person and is quite a good listener. She carries the burdens of five children and their children with grace and equilibrium. I know now what the generations have relied on, a mother's true love and perseverance.

Amber is beginning to lose her hair again. That statement puts fear in me. She came in to my bedroom and I tried to console her, allowing her to show her feelings and validating them. It's the best thing I can do. I can't fix it. I'm all fixed out. This is unfair and I know it and she knows it, but all we can do together is accept the inevitable. Once it is all out, she will be able to do that as before. I never knew this before, but losing over 25 hairs per brushing is above normal. That tidbit can be put in the round file.

Can I honestly tell her "It's going to be all right?" I tried that before the last C.A.T. scan results sent her into a two-week depression. I don't want to set her up for that again. What I can to is keep her in today and remind her to experience what goodness today can bring and not obsess over what may happen tomorrow.

Chapter Thirty-one

Realization, infiltration, aggravation, anticipation

Friday, October 13, 1995

It's been two weeks since I last wrote. I can finally reflect on my feelings. In this last two weeks I've finished my midterms and I truly think I cannot continue with school. My heart is not in it, my brain isn't either. The days of the importance of getting a Bachelor's degree are over. I have a much more important degree to earn, the degree of a cure for my daughter. She needs me more than I need an education. This was just the next step towards my duty to stay busy when my children grew up and left the nest. The nest is still full and needs a mama.

The decision did not come out of a sense of guilt. It came after Amber's chemotherapy infiltrated the tissue of her left arm. The persistence of her doctor, determined to administer therapy, despite five attempts to get a vein to cooperate, went out into her flesh when the vein collapsed. He monitored her closely, pushing the Mustard (chemotherapy drug) in himself to make sure it wasn't leaking. Her arm began to swell. I knew forcing this had been a mistake, but it was too late.

These chemicals are known to be able to penetrate tile on the floor if dropped on it. Imagine how it felt as it burned up her skin from the inside out. Within two days her arm was red, swollen and burning. We tried ice packs, hot packs, Tylenol. Nothing helped. Finally a Vicodine gave her some relief. It took eleven days before she could go without a painkiller. There is a knot in her skin, the infected area about the size of her hand is dark red and is no longer soft as the rest of her skin surrounding the area.

I am mad as hell and I can't say a thing. Technically, Amber is the patient and since she is 18, I have no chance to meet with the doctor to ask questions or speak my mind. I realized that when I tried before to address the issue of the last C.A.T. scan. I am scared if I become the enemy, he would refuse to treat her. My hands are tied. Amber needs to have trust in her doctor, and if she doesn't want to call him on this, I cannot do it for her.

Sunday, October 29, 1995

It's been an up and down week. Amber scared me on Thursday when she told me about a lump she felt on her groin area and also tenderness under her armpit. I went into a weird tailspin. Bridgett was with me and witnessed her mom falling apart emotionally. I cried and got out all the pamphlets I had on Hodgkin's disease, which showed the lymph node pattern on the body. I ran with this, couldn't see straight, and I'm not sure how I managed to get us to the doctor's office, but I did. I barely maintained sanity long enough to get this there. Bridgett was also upset and crying. How could this be happening? No way.

Finally, he examined Amber and said it was just an inflamed hair follicle. Meanwhile, I was picking up the pieces of my brain and heart that had shattered everywhere. When I began breathing again, two hours later, all he did was tickle her unmercifully, gave her some antibiotics and sent her on her way. Talk about a false alarm. Thank God.

Her next C.A.T. scan is November 10th. I am going to try to stay neutral on this one, which is a hard thing to do. Which path will Amber's be?

Chapter Thirty-two

<u>Share the good news</u>

Monday, November 13, 1995

    Yesterday was the happiest day of my life! Amber has beaten her cancer. Dr. Dan came to the park where we were having a benefit Bar-B-Q for Elena Macedo's up coming bone marrow transplant, and told her she was "done." As they sat together in the shade of the trees with purple and white balloons bouncing about their heads, he gave her the great news. She is done with chemo. This is a great day! I was cleaning up garbage and walking around, not noticing or even remotely thinking why Dr. Dan would be there. He waited until he was alone with Amber and then casually said, "Well, I'll bet you will be happy because you are done." She thought he was referring to the raffle tickets she was selling, when it clicked, she began to cry, then they hollered for me to come over. I thought we had won the raffle. Instead we won something much bigger. Amber's freedom.

    I have been telling people the good news ever since and it just keeps getting better. Amber has beaten it! We all have beaten it with the help of our Higher Power fighting off the evil one. It almost seems unreal I must pinch myself. It has been a long haul. That dark cloud that hovered over me is almost gone. All the doubts and fears and anxiety have been replaced by hope for the present and future. I could write a book.

Chapter Thirty-three

Easing back to normalcy

Saturday, November 25, 1995

We are resting after a long day at the San Diego Zoo. It was so much fun and the weather was beautiful. We all are getting along and we have a reason to celebrate—Amber's remission.

We spent Thanksgiving driving to Donna's home in San Juan Capistrano. The dinner was great and we were able to share our good news with close friends. However, I have decided I want to begin having the turkey dinner tradition at our own home from now on.

The hotel is marvelous. Could it be we are all so thankful a barn would be ok, too? The girls are playing cards and Tom is reading the sports page of the local paper. We went to a movie last night and haven't done that in so long it was fun. Just being together as a family out of crisis is the best part of it all.

The last time we were here as a family, we were bringing Amber here to USD for her first semester away from home. That seems like eons ago. I am still going to miss my girl when she goes back for the winter semester, and she is very excited about that. I have to admit I'm not there yet, but I have vowed to support her in any way I can. She deserves to be where she wants to be. She is with us now and that's all that matters.

Monday, November 27, 1995

The trip home was uneventful although there was lots of traffic. We just got settled in when Amber came out of her bedroom in tears. She had absent-mindedly felt along her incision scar on her neck and discovered a small bump about the size of a pea. I tried to convince her that this was not anything to worry about, but the fear was etched on her face. I finally had to give her some Calms relaxant to help her go to sleep.

The next day we saw Dr. Dan, and he put her mind at ease by saying it was a "whatzit," his term for nothing to worry about. She breathed a deep sigh of relief and all was ok again.

On my way to town the next day, I prayed my finger rosary (holding onto the steering wheel and counting Hail Mary's on my fingers) all the way to my destination. Some concern and "what if" crept up on me. So this is Amber's life from now on. We will have to accept it. I have to accept a lot of things. Like her going back to college in February. I better live in today and enjoy her while I can. Meanwhile Bridgett keeps us hopping. She is now without a car. We took it away from her for ditching second period without my knowledge. Never a dull moment, a constant reminder that life goes on.

Meanwhile, I am gearing up for my finals. And I mean finals. I won't be going back to school for a while. Once I get through my last final before Christmas, that's it for me. I want to enjoy the holidays and celebrate our gratitude of Amber's continued remission.

Even though money is tight, we have to make the next month extra special. The time Tom took off to be home is taking its toll. The only times he was able to stay home from work was for major procedures or C.A.T. scan results. The rest of the time he had to be in San Francisco where the work was plentiful. Being away from his little girl was very hard on him. In the construction trade you have to go where the work is and no pay is subsidized if you aren't on the job. He worked just enough hours to keep our health insurance. The cost for all those tests, procedures, labs, chemotherapy, transfusions, etc. would have put us in the poor house without insurance.

The benefit for Elena was for just that reason. Their insurance company would not approve her bone marrow transplant. As it turned out, they raised enough money to help, but without insurance these expenses could break them. Elena is only five years old and she was diagnosed at the age of four. That family has gone through hell. When Amber and Elena met for the first time they clicked. Even though their ages are many years apart they have become good buddies. Our families have clung together through good and bad. Meeting at the American Cancer Societies " Camp Reach for the Stars," in June was one of the best things that ever happened to us. I don't know very much about the type of cancer Elena has, but it is in the family of Wilm's tumors, and I know that she has had to have one of her kidneys removed.

Amber is in awe of this little champion. They both have been through so much, but at the age of six it's got to be hard to comprehend. I'm an adult and I have trouble. Is innocence what we need to get through it all?

C   atastrophic
A   ltering life
N   o fair
C   onsuming
E   rratic
R   evolting

This black dark hole
It's endless core
Swallows us whole
No life as before
Robs young and old
Fills us with dread
Places much doubt
Inside my head

Janine
5/96

Chapter Thirty-four

Cruising along

Saturday, December 16, 1995

Another visit with Dr. Dan confirmed his first opinion of the mysterious lump on her neck. He still says it is nothing to be concerned about. Amber is skittish, and that is to be expected. After all, it has only been a month since he pronounced her "done."

I told him about her going back to college at USD and he said it was the best thing for Amber. It's time for her to be with her young friends and have some fun. On a serious note, we saw Erin at the office while we were there and she was receiving intravenous pain meds for her throat. The radiation has made it so unbearable to swallow she has lost a lot of weight. Robin and Don were there with her. They looked so empty. I was taken back to my own days in that room with Amber for similar tortures. Like stepping into a nightmare. We could wake up this time and walk out of that office. Erin has to continue to live the nightmare.

As if seeing Erin wasn't enough to upset us all, we received a call from Tom's mother. Cancer strikes again. The tumors are around her liver. No treatment has been ordered. I don't understand why, but she is 70 years old. Maybe they think her quality of life would be better to opt out of chemo. I don't know what to think. They are so far away. Now the shoe is on the other foot, so to speak. I hate to admit it, but I'm very glad Amber's shoes are brand new.

Amber and Bridgett cried. This hit Amber harder after having been through her own battle. It's a sad thing all the way around, but at least she knows what her enemy is at last. When they were here she had lost so much weight and complained of pain and being sick so much. So, we pray and that's about all we can do.

Chapter Thirty-five

Rebirth, rejoice, recover

Thursday, December 28, 1995

I'm about to bring in the new year of 1996 and all I can say is it couldn't get any worse than '95.

A lot happened after my last entry, (August 8th) but I chose not to write in my journal because it became harder to have to write down the incidents. Almost like having to re-live my experiences. I couldn't do it.

It turned out in August that I was told that therapy wasn't finished and that I would have to complete another two months of therapy. If the mass stayed the same that time I would be done. I had counted so much on being done in six months that the thought of continuing was unbearable. The news devastated me. All I wanted was to get back to my "normal" life. What ever that was!

After a couple of weeks of depression I finally accepted my fate. I was to committed to 15 units at Hancock and nervous that I wouldn't be able to hang while still going through "chemo", but I challenged myself anyway. In the meantime me and my Mom joined Weight Watchers and began my struggle for self-improvement. I swore that the set back of treatment wasn't going to continue to rule my self-esteem.

Currently I have lost 14 lbs. I originally weighed in at 138 and presently weigh 123.

My new goal is 120. (I've given up my dream of my high school weight.)

Regardless of therapy, life improved for me in those couple months. My hair was at a cute length and it didn't fall out like I thought it might. I started school looking fairly normal and people were shocked when they discovered I was still on chemo. In this time of rebirth I really started to set my priorities. My health and family were first, then good grades and academics then social aspects. God was above all because he made it all possible for me.

By the time for my C.A.T. scan I went into it with a whole different outlook. I didn't allow myself to get my hopes up and I was willing to accept whatever the results might be. This time I was prepared. I had the C.A.T. scan on Friday and once again had to wait for the results over the weekend. (Talk about stress) Luckily me and my family were helping with a benefit for a five year old named Elena Macedo who went to Camp Reach for the Stars with me and was due to have a bone marrow transplant. I felt really good about helping with such a good cause and sold raffle tickets at the BBQ. When Dr. Dan showed up I wasn't surprised because he, too, had donated to the cause. (Along with being my doctor he was also the camp doctor) He sat next to me and casually started some random conversation as usual and did so for about 15 min. Finally, after I had mentioned how I happy I was for the wonderful turnout when he asked me how happy I would be to know I was done. I had no idea what he was talking about. And for a moment I thought he meant about selling the raffle tickets. Casually he mentioned that he had reviewed my results early and that I was done with treatment. I have never been so shocked by anything in my whole life!

This was on Sunday, Nov. 12th. A day of which I will never forget. Not many doctors would take the time on a Sunday afternoon to deliver such news that could have waited until Monday. Dr. Dan is a very special doctor and friend to me. I would have never met him without my misfortune, but it happened for a reason and I am thankful. Through my rough year I have been touched by many and am happy to say that I, too, have touched others. On that very special Sunday in November I touched the hearts of the Macedo family. My good news brought them hope for their daughters rough journey ahead and happiness in a time of fear. They call me Elena's Angel because I gave her the strength and courage to face her upcoming challenge. She looks at my victory as a sign that she, too, will beat it.

Somewhere…

Somewhere there's a place for

me.

Where I'm always wanting

to be.

Somewhere all of my dreams

will come true.

Where I'll never have to be blue.

Somewhere I'll find a love

again

whom will be loving and

my best friend.

Somewhere I'll fit in perfectly

I'll never have to stop

being me

There's a place out there

waiting for me.

One day I will find it

just you wait and see.

Amber Carter

Chapter Thirty-six

Forgiveness means freedom

Friday, December 29, 1995

I find it easier to motivate myself to write in my journal now. Whether it is because I'm not always writing about depressing things or just have more energy, I think it's for the better. Now I can write about good things and bad things that are now in the past with a better out-look.

Tonight I experienced something that I expected to happen yet was a big step for me. Monica called me and asked me to a movie and coffee. This was the first phone call from her since this time last year. With mixed feelings I agreed to go. Forgiveness is going to be the hardest in my time of recovery because I've had so many friends who turned their backs on me when I needed them most. And now when it's all over they want to be friends again when they won't have to deal with the "C" word.

I agreed to go tonight because Monica had the guts to admit that she was wrong the other day when I ran into her. She admitted that her drug problem was the excuse of her change yet it was no excuse. She realized that it was very selfish of her and that she had felt awful about it for some time. This whole apology took place at her work and was incorporated with tears. I never pressured her for what she said, I only mentioned that it had been a "tough" year. (Wasn't that an understatement!?!)

This whole incident really made me think. In the days following, before her call, I real-

ly evaluated whether or not I should forgive her or rather "if" I could. The answer was yes. If she had the guts to humble herself and admit she was wrong, I could give her a second chance, yet I knew that first I had to tell her how I felt.

Tonight after the movie we went out for coffee and tried to summarize all we had been through since we last talked. Eventually she asked me how I felt about her as a friend. I was completely honest, and in tears I explained to her how hard it had really been to lose all of my friends including her.

We both cried and got a lot off of our chests and at the end of our talk we both felt 100% better about it. Forgiveness is a beautiful thing. I never thought I would be able to forgive anyone who let me down, but I proved myself wrong tonight. Trust will have to be rebuilt and I explained to her that we'll have to start all over, but friendship will be possible. We both are two different people because of our experiences and I hope it works out.

Chapter Thirty-seven

<u>Goodbye to 1995,</u>
<u>Don't let the door hit you in the ass</u>

Sunday, December 31, 1995
   The last day of 1995. I can't say I'm sad to see it go. It has been a dreadful year, filled with anxiety, fear, and uncertainty. It's been very hard to keep on going, watching Amber suffer, lose her hair, gain weight, be so isolated and without friends. It's been a heartbreaking year, an emotional one. Enough emotions to last a lifetime. Hard on our life as a family unit—sometimes the tension threatened to break it apart.
   The dark cloud of cancer filled my every waking moment, stretching my faith in God and the unfairness of it all. It has been a year of alienation between Bridgett and "the Big Three." Turning towards her friends for comfort and denying her feelings of resentment and anger. We have suffered through surgeries, pokes, second opinions, tests, scans, biopsies, inadequate insurance referrals, personal differences and down right cruelness on the part of some medical staff.
   I know how to read the pain on Amber's face even when she would tell me, "It's OK, Mom." Her illness overshadowed every trip, every plan, every single weekend. It's been on my mind, in my heart and in my gut since the fateful night we sat in the car in the parking lot at Dr. Steward's office, raining inside and outside as Amber said, "I don't want to die!"

Along with the inevitable chemotherapy treatments, we met some caring, wonderfully, optimistic nurses and caretakers, and to say the most about our stupendous, humorous and outrageous Dr. Dan. He is the best.

The heartwarming stream of well wishing letters and cards from Aunt Camille—"Life with Lauren." Amber brought out the best in family and friends along with their kind words and prayers abounding. The greatest Camp Reach for the Star's, where we made life-long friendships with other families affected by cancer. We met parents that were in the same boat as us, struggling to make sense of it all. Asking each other the questions, Why, how? Receiving support of those who went before us and survived and the hope of those in remission.

Life tried to go on. I started Cal Poly, Bridgett hung by a thread in some classes, out of school a lot by choice. Tom miraculously kept his job at Diablo Canyon power plant for an entire year and is still going strong, providing us with the excellent insurance for the best possible care for Amber. He plugged along day after day to meet our financial needs, but still getting further into debt than ever. The expenses were great this year. Extras to help us all cope with the gripping fear of dealing with cancer of our loved one. Trips to get our minds off of it, and a trip to get a second opinion. Expenses included: new bedroom furniture and television for Amber, alternative medicines, and painkillers, medical co-payments, a wig, special shampoos for hair loss, special foods to increase appetite, immune boosting vitamins. Things the average family doesn't have to include in their budget. What's a budget?

Through it all, our first concern was to get the best for Amber. It was her welfare and positive outlook that spurred us on. That ever-present smile and hugs that could melt my heart.

That glorious day Dr. Dan came to Elena's benefit and shared the wonderful news of Amber's end of the agony of chemotherapy and the fact that she was cancer free. We were surrounded by our friends who cared and wished her well.

Now the healing begins. 1996 is the year of a new beginning. I hope Amber gets that special kiss tonight that gives her the butterflies in her tummy and proves to her she is wanted, attractive, young, and WELL! I hope Bridgett can resist the boys a little better, that she sees her self worth, not through sexual intentions of some loser.

I just want my girls to be happy with a boy who loves them and will cherish them, the way my husband loves me.

Chapter Thirty-eight

The winds of change

Sunday, January 14, 1996

     I have decided to get enrolled for the winter quarter at Poly. With Amber going back to USD this month, I am going to throw myself back into school. Bridgett is still being a typical teenage rebel, so I can't see my relationship with her improving until Amber leaves and she is an only child again. Meanwhile she is dating a boy we do not approve of. This guy treats her badly and is not a good influence. She is pushing all the buttons possible to alienate us from her. I know adolescence is tough, but this is wearing on me.

     I finally convinced the entire family to go and have some portraits done. It is something we haven't done since we moved to California seven years ago. Now with Amber going away again I am feeling like a family outing is in order. Since location pictures are very expensive, I loaded up my tripod and 35 millimeter camera and we headed down to Shell Beach. The day was perfect. No wind, the sun was out and the ocean sparkling. We had a picnic lunch first and even though Bridgett did her share of grumbling she finally came around when I started shooting pictures of her and her sister. This is a memory maker and we needed a positive shove in that direction. As a family we haven't done anything that involved talking and doing something besides watching television. The tension was broken between Bridgett and her dad over the new boyfriend and we bonded as a family. It was a most memorable day.

The evening left Tom and I alone as Amber and Sandra went out together and Bridgett joined her friends as well. It was nice. Soon, we will be alone a lot. Only two more weeks and Amber goes away to college. I have to remind myself to stay in today.

Monday, January 15, 1996

The days are clicking by. Time is going too fast. I want to savor these next days before Amber leaves. She went to Santa Barbara on Friday to be with Sandra and came back tired and grumpy. She said she missed her own bed. I hope she will be comfortable in her dorm when she goes to USD. She seems to be strong one minute and fragile the next.

School is winding up for me. I'm engulfed with material to read and feel like I find little time to do anything else recreational. However, I'm glad that I will have school to keep me busy when Amber goes away. I need the distraction and what better thing than lots of homework and projects to do.

Meanwhile, Tom finally talked to Bridgett about his opinion of her new boyfriend. I don't know how it went as they talked privately, but Bridgett seemed more stand-offish and also still makes snide comments about the situation under her breath. I can hear her mocking her dad's comments. Obviously it was not a successful bonding experience. It's very tense around here, but Amber and I made a pact to stay out of it and assertively tell them both to talk about their anger to one another, not involve us. That elephant sure knows how to crap in our living room.

Amber has been on edge since getting back from Santa Barbara. She seems to be preoccupied most of the time. I know the situation with her sister and dad is not helping matters, but I still wonder if there is something she is not telling me. Could it be that she is having second thoughts about going away to school? Hadn't she mentioned the possibility of finishing her general education classes at Hancock and then transferring back to USD for her upper division? Time will tell. She's bound to reach a point of conversation soon. After all, the wheels are in motion for her to attend college there this semester. We will be taking her down there on the 27th. Our reservations are already made at the Days Inn in San Diego.

Chapter Thirty-nine

<u>The Beast rears its ugly head</u>

Friday, January 19, 1996

Today I met with Dr. Dan because my anxiety just couldn't go on any longer. The lump that he called "scar tissue" just doesn't seem normal. For the past few weeks I have experienced stiff necks and unexplainable pains and I finally decided to go see the doctor one last time before I leave for college next weekend. After all, recurrence is always on my mind and having a lump with pain doesn't make it any easier to ignore until my C.A.T. scan in March.

So I went by myself to discuss what is "normal" to chemo patients after they are done. Obviously damage was done all over the body but I wondered if pain was normal. I started to cry immediately just talking to him about my fears. I've been worried for a while now and feelings have really been stuffed. Finally I asked him to feel the lump one more time. He was quiet and felt around for a long time while I jabbered and made excuses for why I might be experiencing pain then he mentioned that he wanted to have me get a needle biopsy of it. He says it's only to put my worries at ease, but I think it's because the lump has grown and he's worried. Right now so many emotions are running through my mind. He said that if it was back I could undergo radiation, but that only scares me worse. I want this whole nightmare to be over. I can't help but think that I had something to do with what's happening to me. For instance if I had only taken better care of myself and not partied or stayed out late. I don't understand why

I always have a crisis going on in my life. One ailment after the next. I feel cursed or something. I must have done something pretty rotten to deserve all of this. I accepted all that went on last year and am able to look at the good in it, but it still was HELL! I don't want to go through that again! I thought I'd got the meaning of it all, the lesson I was supposed to get. I'm a new person because of it but I don't have the strength to do it again!

BOOK THREE

DAYS OF HOPE

Days of Hope
Away from home
Once again
All I want to do
Is be well
Tell Bridgie I love her
Don't worry, mom
Love, Amber
~This is a good day to live~

Chapter One

Please take this cup from me

Monday, January 22, 1996

     Well, a year ago on this same Monday I had the same needle aspiration that I had today and once again at 4:30 pm this afternoon I received the same shocking news. To my surprise in the time of the last three months my Hodgkin's disease has recurred. Once again I can't go back to USD after all. The plans have been made including the hotel room for next weekend. My world has again been turned upside down. Except this time things are a bit more serious. Since my cancer came back so soon there is a possibility that I may need to undergo a bone marrow transplant. Dr. Dan thinks that my cancer is partially resistant to MOPP/ABV and a new approach must be taken. Despite the shocking news I've been amazingly calm I guess I expected and prepared myself for the news. Of course I cried a little after seeing my parents' reaction, but I've been the strongest out of all of us. I guess I just feel ready for anything after the hell I've already been through. I don't know what's ahead but in a strange sort of way I know it is going to be ok.

     Tomorrow is the C.A.T. scan, which will help to determine what type of treatment will be necessary, but until then I'm going to be positive and strong.

Wednesday, January 24, 1996

I can hardly put into words what I feel. Amber is no longer cancer free, and she probably never was. This disease is the devil's work I'm sure of it. It is a conniving, evil lurking around her body. She knew it was back from the first time she felt the lump. All the poking and prodding of her doctor saying it's a "whatzit" didn't convince her. It never did.

She has been worried about it since it first raised its ugly head. I wasn't prepared for what Dr. Dan would say. Postpone college. I expected more of a pat on the back, a kiss on the cheek and to wish her Godspeed.

There is a new fear creeping in on my mind. If eight treatments didn't get rid of it, what will? What the hell is a bone marrow transplant? If it is anything like the bone marrow biopsies, I'm really scared. We are back to the unknown. Knowing the effects of MOPP/ABV chemo and the fact that it only pissed the cancer cells off, what is she in for next?

The hospital of choice is City of Hope. We've been there, done that and didn't like it. It is big and impersonal and looks too much like a place for sick people. Amber doesn't belong there. She belongs back in college with her cute hairdo, new lease on life and so on. What happened, God? What the hell happened?

I need to learn lessons from my child. She has an attitude of strength and perseverance and most of all, acceptance. We have been receiving phone calls from everyone. Concerned friends and family are in shock. Only two and a half months of respite for her. They are in disbelief. So are we. But Amber is not. She is handling the calls much better this time. In fact, I see such a strength and acceptance in her that was never there before. As if she is resigned to this fate. Not many tears have been shed by her, some new fears, but she is taking them in stride and isn't saying "Why me?" It's as if she is girding herself for battle.

Amber has an appointment with Dr. Spyberg at the City of Hope in six days. This will be a consultation for treatment plans that will be decided by the end of the following week. Waiting, wondering, worrying.

Tuesday, January 29, 1996

Our little friend, Elena, was in the hospital getting a blood transfusion so Amber and I decided to go by and have a visit with her. When we got there this precious five year-old was propped up in bed, plugged into the machine with a tube connecting her to a bag of blood. She was receiving the products through her Hickman, a catheter placed surgically, to prepare her for the bone marrow transplant that will take place shortly, hopefully. Awaiting the blood that would help make her feel better, she was busily playing with her new Barbie doll and her pony she named Rainbow. Remarkable. Her mom, and my dear friend Julie, says Elena still shows cancer in her pelvis and if it doesn't clear up with chemo, they won't do the BMT. What a world—hard to know what to pray for. I'm praying Amber won't need one and Julie's praying Elena will get the chance to have one.

While we were there, Elena showed Amber her Hickman. It is a catheter surgically placed under the skin with a tube hanging out of it with a split into two. It is the one requested for the BMT by the physicians. It has a "dual port." Whatever that means. I'm sure we will find out. On the way home Amber was very quiet. I sensed her trying to gradually accept the inevitable. It's not like picking out the right color of blouse to buy. This stuff is serious. There is an unknown element that makes me uneasy. I'm praying for strength to get me to a place of understanding. More than that I'm asking God for knowledge of his will for Amber.

Chapter Two

<u>Stream of consciousness</u>

Wednesday, January 31, 1996

It's 5:30 am, been up since 4:30. I can't sleep. My heart beats wildly, I don't know why. I have a sense of urgency with no place to go. I have so much ticking away in my mind lying in bed, and then I get up and there's nothing to do. I feel very small and insignificant, forgotten by God. I have resentments about the way things are going. It's unfair to the point of screaming. I'd like to hide, but there is no place to go.   I want to wake up and discover I've been having a nightmare and everything is ok. I wake up and realize this is the nightmare. When I'm awake I'm exhausted, when I go to sleep I wake up suddenly panicked, like I have so much to do. I just want the comfort of my mother, but that wouldn't even be enough. I want something big and fluffy and warm to hug me and let me cry all I want. I want it to tell me it's gonna' be all right and it will take care of me. I want to feel secure and in control. I feel out of control. I want to watch the horizon and quietly make plans for a future of peace and serenity.

Monday, February 5, 1996

On Friday I had to go to City of Hope to have another bone marrow biopsy which, despite Demerol, (painkiller) still hurt horribly. At least I had my Mom there to hold my hand

and calm me. My butt is sure sore even after three days.

I haven't received any results from my blood or bone marrow tests, but I have heard that I'm scheduled for radiation therapy next Monday at City of Hope. I hope this means that everything checked out ok. My Mom and I will have to live at City of Hope while I undergo radiation every day for about two weeks, then if all goes well I will begin the BMT procedure.

I'm scared, but for some reason I'm remarkably strong. I believe it is God who is helping me be this way. I just know that all of this needs to be done, and with God's help I can get through anything. I pray each night for his strength and help and continue to have faith that he hears me.

I don't know what's ahead, but through all that I've been through I know that I appreciate and treasure today!

Sometimes it's tough not to project into the future and dwell in my misfortunes, but in doing so I am nothing but frustrated and upset. By focusing on the hear and now I am able to be happy and enjoy my time with my family. They are the most important people in my life!

Saturday, February 10, 1996

Well, tomorrow I head down to City of Hope to begin my radiation treatments, which will supposedly last two weeks. Tonight I'm feeling very emotional and scared. I fear that this is a last hope for me and I pray that it works. My Dad and sister will stay home while me and my Mom will stay there. I was sitting in my room tonight looking at what I will be missing and beings that the wheels will soon be in motion I wonder if I will see them for a long time. I guess my biggest fear is that I will go through all of this horrible stuff and will end up dying anyway. I don't want to die and don't even want to think about it, but sometimes it pops up in the back of my mind "what if..."

So tonight I look at my family, my cat, my room, my house, and wonder "what if..." these are the last times that I will see you. This thought makes me very scared, sad, not to mention how I will miss everyone and everything when I'm away.

I pray to God that I am doing the right thing and soon all of this hard work and faith will pay off. But it is very difficult to let all of my worries go, and let God take care of things. I pray that tomorrow I leave with courage and the faith to get through whatever will come in the next few months.

Thursday, February 8, 1996

The week is drawing to a close quickly. I have been busy making arrangements for Amber and I to go to Hope Village to stay while she has daily radiation treatments. She is finally showing some signs of fear and anxiety. She cried with me last night, telling me some hard realities that obviously have been wearing on her. What if this doesn't work? A dark thought I've had myself. No hope for having her own eggs intact after full body radiation. A thought like that has crept into mind lately. These are way too serious, up there with the worst of them—all those nightmares we have and wake up and it's a just a dream—well, this one's real. I can't let this happen and I won't. I will remain hopeful and know that for every closed door, one new one will be opened.

I sometimes slip out of myself and look back and am shocked. If I were to hear news of someone else's child having a relapse and become a candidate for bone marrow transplant, I would be freaked out. What would I say? Those shallow things I hear from people like, "I'll pray for you, I'm thinking of you, I'll be there for you, is there anything I can do." All the BS that "normies" say and then go home to their happy little families and jobs and school and future. They don't have a clue. I would rather have them be silent and admit they don't know <u>what </u>to say. How could anyone possible "understand?" So I'm dropping that word from my vocabulary.

Chapter Three

<u>Love, laugh, live</u>

Sunday, February 11, 1996

Our last day home before we travel down south to Duarte, CA where the hospital sits quietly nestled in a rose garden of undeterminable size. If I didn't know better, I'd think we were at a state park instead of a major medical center. I guess the flowers are supposed to calm the savage reason for being there, but once those automatic doors open at the entrance you are gobbled up in the frazzled world of life-threatening disease.

I made the necessary phone calls for preparation for our stay at what they lovingly call Hope Village. Or is it Village of the Damned? Oops, a little Freudian slip there. I can let that happen in the privacy of my dear friend, the journal, but keep it our secret opinion. It's just that ever since the news of Amber's recurrence, there seems to be a deep unspoken fear in our family. A fear only sardonic humor can help me make sense of. If you ever witnessed a meeting with Julie and I, you would see us laugh at the most awful things like, "How to use Emla cream before plucking your eyebrows." (a topical anesthetic for numbing before an injection) Or even better, a look at the world of kids with cancer, Erma Bombeck's book, *I wanna Grow Hair, I wanna Grow up, I wanna go to Boise*. This takes place at a summer cancer camp. The camp directors wanted her to write about how cancer, chemo treatments, and loss of hair fits wonderfully well and quite as normal as any other summer camp for kids. An example at our own Camp Reach for the Stars held in the first week of June in Cambria, Ca was a boy who put sunscreen the shape of a happy face on the top of his baldhead. You can imagine the results. Awesome.

Humor is the only way we all stay sane. There is a sad bit of irony to that statement, the most serious of diseases, a real killer, ends up making you insane enough to laugh at odd things that make well people shudder.

While I ramble, our friends Julie, Greg, and Elena are at a crossroads with her treatment options. They are at Stanford Medical Center near San Francisco where they still await the news of possible BMT for her. What began as a fundraiser for their family, and happiness beyond belief for ours turned out to be the last really happy time we shared with them. Now this five year old will be Amber's inspiration, and her parents will be mine.

We saw Erin at the doctor's office on Friday. She was so pale, thin, and bald with no life in her eyes. Will that be Amber in a month? It's so hard to think about that now. We will do what needs to be done and eradicate this thing once and for all.

Chapter Four

<u>The Mask</u>

Monday, February 12, 1996

    We settled in at the Village and Amber had to immediately report to the radiation department. It was an excruciating day for Amber, as she had to be prepped for the actual radiation treatment that will take place tomorrow. She had to lay on a simulator table while three doctors stepped over each other to take care of her properly. Dr. Robodek is her radiation oncologist. He is also the head of research and takes very few patients. He made it clear that Amber was important because C.O.H. needed success for their studies. He was tactful about it, but the message was clear that she has the best chance here to get well for selfish business reasons as well as humane ones. Her young age and vitality is a plus and for whatever reason they are doing everything in their power to cure her, I'm all for it.

    Amber looked like a sheet of graph paper, a grid of blue ink and red fluorescent laser cross marks from her head to her sternum and across from shoulder to shoulder. The room was cold, they covered her with a warmed blanket, but it did little to help warm her nerves and mine. It was like stepping into a Star Trek movie set. I pulled a chair up and sat as close to her as they would allow, but I could only watch. I couldn't rub her feet, soothe her brow or cover her breasts that were exposed. It was horribly unsettling.

I tried to talk to the doctor's and tell them about Amber, the person, not the patient. I was clearly out of my league. They just kept pushing buttons and doing math calculations from behind a window looking out into the room where Amber's still body lay open to see. To make matters worse they had to make a mask from some type of plastic cheesecloth type material that they warmed up and formed over her face. With her eyes and mouth closed they pulled it tight over her face and attached it to the table. She looked like a mummy. It was an eerie sight, but I knew she was inside the cocoon, trying to be brave, laying there on the table, all alone. This is a lonely disease. I try to be there for her but the strength has to come from within her somehow.

She managed to maintain her dignity while being exposed to the doctors. She knew what she had to do, but being so young and innocent, she must have felt so vulnerable lying there. My heart aches for what she had to endure. I hope tomorrow isn't so challenging or traumatic. Most of all, I wish I could take her place.

The radiation of the tumor behind her sternum has to be exact. Since the heart and lungs are there, painstaking figures are necessary. There were at least six different technicians doing their separate calculations and pooling their information collectively. That information will be used to make a lead plate to go over the major organs and protect them and still allow the radiation to get the difficult location of the tumor. This culprit is not the only concern; there are nodes in her lungs that the rest of the high dose chemotherapy will annihilate. Once the radiation is completed, that will begin. I don't know much more at this point. I am learning all about these highly technical procedures as we go along. It's easy to see how overwhelming it would be to try and comprehend it all at once. And no one at this point has even tried to explain the whole thing to us anyway. The medical personnel who know everything are too busy, and the ones back home only have a clue.

Bone marrow transplants, autogolous and analogous, stem cell transplants, collection, and harvest of stem cells. These are specialized and the latest chosen way to beat the crap out of resistant cancer cells. The only other new ways are in clinical trials, many hundreds of them. Amber and I just read, look up stuff on the computer when we can, contact the Johnson's and the Macedo's and try to pool our own information with what is the cutting edge of cancer warfare at the moment. It helps me to learn about the beast and possible ways to tame or kill it. On the other hand, Tom prefers to remain unenlightened.

Chapter Six

__Put out the fires, mom__

Tuesday, February 13, 1996

 Last night Bridgett called me crying. She misses me, couldn't sleep and sounded quite helpless. She tries to be so grown up and strong; it's a rare occasion when she acts helpless. It is a scary thing to be left without your mom and knowing your sissy is going through some bizarre treatment that you don't even understand. I talked to her for a while and sensed her finally calming down. She has another head cold and that doesn't help. I hate seeing our family split apart, but there's no other way to do this. This is a time when I wish my mom were around to take up the slack. We are a thousand miles away from that possibility. I shudder to think when we are here for a month during the transplant. That will be even harder as Tom will be working a lot of overtime next month that he can't afford to pass up if he wants to keep his job. What do we do? Maybe one of my sisters can come out for a visit and be a surrogate mom for a month. It is too early to plan anything, but I can put it out there.

Wednesday, February 14, 1996

 This is our third day at Hope Village. Yesterday was another busy one on the simulator for Amber. She shared with me that she was very upset the first day of The

Mask. I knew it had been hard, but I had no idea how devastated she was. The guilt began to rise in me as she spoke.

"I feel like I have been raped." She was crying softly. My heart was breaking. "They put that thing on my face and I couldn't move, see, or talk. I could barely breathe as if someone was holding my mouth closed. Then the blanket was pulled down and my boobs were just out there for all those men to see. I was humiliated." She kept crying as I held her hand. "No one knows how I felt. I was frozen and couldn't even cry or scream or ask you to cover me up."

How could I have been so blind? My daughter had been treated like a piece of meat on a slab and I just sat there and watched. Why?

"I'm so sorry, Amber." My stomach was turning at the thought of what she had been through. From her perspective she felt like she had been viciously violated. From this one incident she felt like a victim and that was not acceptable.

"What can we do to make it better?" I questioned her sympathetically.

"I don't know, but I have to go back there again and I don't want to."

I was thinking. Here we were, seemingly at the mercy of a strange crowd of doctors, nurses, and technicians. It was a huge hospital; some of the best surgeons and cancer specialists in the U.S. were here. They had probably been doing this simulation thing for years the exact same way. It was a daunting task indeed. I pondered. I knew no one well enough to seek advice.

"Let's write a letter."

At that very moment, I took out paper and we sat there and composed the most heartfelt poison pen letter I'd ever written. In it we explained how Amber had felt so violated and numb from the experience. We wrote for the rest of the afternoon, and then I sealed it in an envelope and put it in Dr. Robodek's box at the hospital, signing it "Anonymous."

With that under her belt, Amber almost seemed triumphant. At least the words were there and no one would be able to persecute her for it since it was not signed. Just a little information that we thought they should have about the human receiving side of procedures. The power of the pen had struck again.

I had written a few of this type of letter since her diagnosis a year ago. One of my favorites was when I wrote to the caseworker assigned to Amber from the health insurance we subscribed to. They had been balking on the approval of the BMT due to the experimental fashion of the procedure. They didn't feel there had been enough proof of its success. Knowing Amber had few options at this point aside from clinical trials, I set my pen to paper. The letter and the picture of Amber I sent to her must have done the trick. They approved the procedure immediately afterwards.

The next time we had to see Dr. Robodek, he mentioned getting an "anonymous" letter in his box. Little did we know, Amber was only one of three patients he had presently. Busted. But, that's ok. He addressed the letter openly and was quite apologetic. He told us that he vowed as a young intern never to let himself become callous with his patients, and admitted to the heinous fact that he had become what he abhorred. Taking this time to speak especially to Amber, he again was reminded to put the patient first, tend their needs, and make their experience as pleasant as possible and even suggested we create an informative pamphlet for future radiation patients.

By putting Amber's feelings on paper we had accomplished two important things. Amber would not settle for anything but respect of her body, and that her feelings mattered. It also gave her some amount of control and took away her role as a victim. Instead, she was able to be a participant in the quest for her cure. And my mission was accomplished to make my daughter the V.I.P. (very important patient) that she was.

Chapter Seven

<u>Vacation from radiation</u>

Thursday, February 15, 1996

    Before her first actual radiation treatment, we took in the sights of Pasadena. Determined to put this out of her mind for a while, I attempted to lighten up our mental load by doing some sight seeing. After all, the radiation treatments only took about 30 minutes and we had the rest of the day free. While Amber still felt good enough, I wanted to get her away from the illness that ruled her life.

    We roamed around Old Town and took in the sunshine and then went to a movie. Afterwards, we found a pleasant little Lebanese restaurant and had dinner. The food was delicious and by the time we got back to the apartment we were ready to retire. I had made the efficiency as cozy as possible. Not knowing what to expect, I brought some throw rugs and placemats for the kitchen area. All other necessities were provided like cooking utensils, dinnerware and silverware, and bedding. I brought a coffee pot and lots of things to snack on. I also brought comforters and Amber's favorite blue afghan. It had been with her for every procedure, transfusion, and chemotherapy treatment back home. We were here for a reason, but it didn't need to feel that way. I pretended this was just the two of us deciding to live together for a while like roommates. But no matter how I tried, even I became lonesome for our own home. This would take some time to adjust to.

Two lab techs would carry out the actual radiation procedure. There was a woman on the team and she was more sensitive to the exposure of Amber's breasts. She drew lines where her lungs and heart were with a permanent marker. Continuing to measure and draw X's, mapping out the areas to be radiated, the special lead plate over-head was attached to the machine and they had to match that up perfectly with the marks they had made on her body.

The radiating area covered her neck where the stubborn disease hid, and into the sternum area where the biggest mass grew. Avoiding any contact with the heart or lungs was the tricky part. But these were trained professionals that knew their jobs. No room for error here.

The mask had to be placed on Amber's face, but she made sure they cut holes for her eyes and mouth. That made it more bearable, even though the mask was attached to the table making movement impossible. To ease the stress they played soothing music in the background to help ease the severity of the situation. In addition to these amenities, they allowed Amber to remove the mask between procedures, sit up and stretch a little before resuming. That's when I could come back into the "vault" and rub her feet, give her water, and a hug, then retreat back to the outside where I kept watch until the sign above the door signaled it was all right to enter.

After Amber received her first treatment she felt tired, achy and sunburned. She said it felt weird when she swallowed, but not necessarily painful. More like discomfort, although her neck is sore and hurting from the position her head is placed inside the mask. At least these lab techs were very personable and empathetic to her and me. (Was it because of the letter? I wondered.)

Sometimes I just can't believe this is happening to her. I look at her and see the worry of things to come on her face. She should be excited about her future, not dread-ing it. She reminisces about her college days at USD then gets down, and I can see her eyes tear up and I know she hates what her life has become and mourns what it could have been.

There were a couple of bright notes in the day. Dr. Dan called and talked to her for a while and made her laugh. She also got a dozen long stemmed roses from the Macedo Family for Valentine's Day. That was a real surprise and lifted her spirits.

We have been taking walks around the hospital grounds. It is truly a beautiful place. They take great pains to keep it that way. There must be a million rose bushes. A statue of Mary is nestled in an alcove in part of the garden, which includes a pond with a waterfall and much foliage. It has a small bench where you can sit and ponder. Get it? A pond to ponder? Gotta' keep my sense of humor. God knows I need it right now. Whatever is happening back home will be waiting for me when I get there. Meanwhile, with her first radiation treatment out of the way, we now have only nine more to go. Soon we will go home for the weekend and get some hometown strokes we greatly need, a vacation from radiation.

Friday, February 16, 1996

Today after Amber's second treatment we met with Karen M., our nurse coordinator, to tour the BMT unit. She will be our contact person to ask questions of and get Amber through this procedure smoothly. She was a wealth of information that answered a multitude of questions from both of us, and she has a kind and gentle manner. It was very helpful to speak to her, and it will make things easier for us to have someone to talk to. This is a big place and I had thought Amber was lost in the shuffle. Until radiation is finished, there is no change of the present plan. More information about what happens next will be given to us later. For now this is enough to digest.

Chapter Eight

<u>Home Sweet Home</u>

Monday, February 19, 1996

     The weekend at home was very nice, but too short. We watched a video on Saturday, Sunday was a family movie after church and some avid card playing—all four of us! Even Bridgett wanted to join in.

     I loved being home, sleeping in my own bed, just being there to clean my own kitchen and have our familiar surroundings. We take far too much for granted the little things we love. Even though the Village is nice and clean, it's not home.

     The trip back down to the hospital was stressful. Between the rain storm and the huge amount of traffic, I ended up doing all the driving. Amber was afraid to drive. I was quite tired and nervous from the trip and all I did was sit for three hours.

Wednesday, February 21, 1996

     It's still raining. We are going to float away! Yesterday was a hassle just going to the grocery store. I have my trusty umbrella so at least we can stay moderately dry, but we didn't bring the right warm clothing. Today after Amber's radiation we'll get out and go shopping.

     We received news from Dr. Robodek that March 11th is a reasonable date for her transplant procedures to begin. Now what will those procedures be? Ok, drop that bomb in your "matter-of-fact-I-know-it-all-you-don't" attitude. Meanwhile, my stomach did a flip. Here we go. I got out the booklet our assigned nurse, Karen, gave us and began to read all about it. I learned a lot of things I didn't want to. Down the road this procedure is going to get scary. Can Amber's body take the punishment? Somehow she must. I feel bewildered at the position she is in and what my role shall be.

This radiation she's getting now and the previous eight months of chemo will seem like a picnic compared to what they have in store for her. For every good thing she will get out of this procedure, there are ten bad side effects. I don't feel equipped intellectually to handle all of this. I'm barely holding it altogether with scotch tape right now. And the hard stuff hasn't even begun…I know how Jesus must have felt when God told him what he had to do. Get nailed to the cross? No way, Jose! I'll pass on that. Can we negotiate on this deal?

This whole thing puts a different perspective on things in my life. Everything looks so small and insignificant in comparison. How important is anything anyway? I feel like I need to be strong way beyond my past experiences with Amber so far. I know she will be near death, as close as anyone will ever be. It scares the crap out of me.

Back at home things are pretty squirrelly. Bridgett's car is on the fritz and Tom has been trying to fix it after work with no luck so far. He has allowed a fellow electrician to stay with them until he can find a place to live. They are both on the same job at the nuke plant and it is time for replacement of the fuel rods. That means lots of overtime, and little time for Bridgett.

I am worried about her. She misses me and is now being thrown into living with only men who talk about work all the time. She needs a clone of me to get her through. What's going to happen when I have to be with Amber during the three weeks it will take for the BMT?

Thursday, February 22, 1996

Amber and I talked at length last night, tucked into our twin beds, as comfy as we possibly could be in a strange environment away from home. She began to cry and I tried to comfort her. Her fears are great. She is afraid she is going to die. How can I listen to this and try to tell her she's wrong when I have had the same dark thoughts myself? I don't want to admit it, but the unknowns of this transplant are putting me on the edge, testing my faith. The "what if's" cloud my mind. I need to pray harder for resolution and strength to help her get through this. I asked her to pray for me and I will pray that we both keep our faith, and optimism.

It is so hard to watch her, now that she looks so healthy and normal on the outside, but inside, but knowing that there is so much wrong. I must shed this doom and gloom. This can be a perfect day if I lead myself through it positively; she will follow as she always does. I shall do that and seize the day—"Carpe Diem!"

Friday, February 23, 1996

It's another sunny day and a good one for traveling home. This will be a short visit as we come back here on Sunday, but we are trying to arrange Angel Flights to take us back on that day. This is an organization of aviators that donate their time and small planes to help patients get to their treatments at hospitals around the U.S. It is a volunteer effort that could save me from driving eight hours to Duarte where City of Hope is located.

We saw Dr. Spyberg yesterday and he said the transplant is definitely the place this journey will take Amber to. More testing has to be done back in our hometown to make sure she is in good enough health to withstand the physical strain this procedure will put her body through. She is having more discomfort from the effects of the radiation. After eight treatments it is becoming difficult to swallow and the diseased lymph nodes in her neck and chest are hurting her as well. She has prescription pain medication, but hates to take Vicodin and Lortab because it makes her constipated and she doesn't like to be "out of it" in her mind. I see her bravely trying to limit herself and the side effects, but the pain is usually too much and she has to resort to taking them as well as some liquid to soothe her throat. Along with these effects, she has heartburn a lot and hiccoughs. She has learned to calm herself enough to get rid of the hiccoughs, mind over matter she says. I wish my mind could get her over all of what's the matter. Finding a form of nourishment has been a challenge. The blender comes in handy, and Ensure keeps her vitamins coming. I need a full time dietician to help me figure this out.

This is just another struggle to beat the disease and the side effects caused to beat it. I have an old nutrition book from one of my pre-requisite college classes that helps explain a lot of the body's blood and vitamin interactions. I'm either reading about the cancer or the effects of treatment on the body or how to boost it to make up for the damage it does to vital organs and blood products. The body is an amazing thing. If you screw around with one thing, you have to take up the slack with something else. There is a constant battle going on for homeostasis. In this instance, there is a foreigner in the hood speaking it's own language and doing its damage without regard to the homies that reside there.

I can't think of anything but this task at hand, to get Amber through this transplant. I've had a lot of mixed feelings—some anger, helplessness, feeling overwhelmed, irritable, apprehension and dread. In some ways I want to know what's next and to get it started. Then I think I'm not ready to start because I must watch Amber suffer. I feel ambivalence between the two evils: the cancer evil and the cancer treatment evil. Her immune system is beginning to nose dive and now a cold has added to her discomfort.

Such things were never included in my dreams for my sweet daughter's future. She should be walking to classes, going to parties, meeting boys, and making new friends. I am so sad this is not true. I have to stay away from these thoughts. We have to get through this for her to live. There will be plenty of days once this is over for her to enjoy. God give me the strength and help me to stay in today.

Chapter Nine

<u>One day at a time</u>

Tuesday, March 5, 1996

There is so much to learn in so little time. This is a crash course in everything we never wanted to know about the world of intravenous options. This was the wave of the future for Amber. She would now have a foreign apparatus in her chest that would guarantee a vein available for the following bombardment of chemotherapy drugs she would be receiving. Also, it would provide a port to receive much needed blood products if she were to become neutropenic, or in need of platelets.

After the surgical placement of the port with two catheter lines that hung out about seven inches from the top of Amber's left breast, we were sent home with some syringes, vials of saline and alcohol solution, gauze, alcohol wipes, swabs, surgical tape, and betadine. All this is needed to flush the tubing that leads to the main artery, the vena cava. When Amber was released from the hospital last night it was terribly late, and I hadn't a clue what to do with all these supplies they sent us home with. No instructions. Just like when she was born 19 years ago.

Thank God for Helen, who again came to our aid this morning and schooled Amber in the art of flushing these lines. This needs to be done daily or she could develop a nasty infection. It is an outside door to the inside of her body and needs to be kept sterile. I watched as Helen instructed Amber in the cleaning and told her that it is always better she takes care of this herself. That way no one else's germs and bacteria would be involved and there would be no unnecessary risk of infection.

While Helen is here instructing Amber, she teaches me the art of giving injections. I am required to administer a shot of GCSF, a blood booster designed to get her stem cells to multiply for the transplant, to Amber daily for the next two weeks. I am very scared I will not be able to do this without hurting her. I pray big time for God to give me strength.

Wednesday, March 6, 1996

I am sitting here in Amber's hospital room at the City of Hope. She is now in her second day of VP16, a combination of 16 different chemotherapy drugs injected in her body through the newly place Hickman catheter lines. This huge amount of drugs is being administered to get her blood count down to wake up the marrow and begin producing more stem cells that will be used for her eventual transplant. Another benefit from this two-day binge on chemotherapy is that these drugs go after and kill the cancer cells living in her lymph nodes. It is amazing that she can even hold up her head under these circumstances. As usual, she has a courageous attitude, and that smile is infectious to the patient next to her. This woman is here for her own special circumstances. Namely breast cancer. We have met so many people and shared their battles. There is no age, gender, race, or monetary background exclusive to those who are stricken with cancer. I would say, however, there are those special ones who choose to remain hopeful. We are in that category.

There is no place for me in the hospital, so we are spending our sleepless nights apart for the first time. Our apartment in the village is dark and gloomy without Amber's company to light it up.   Coming back in the morning I see her finally sleeping after the nurse said she had not gotten any rest through the night. Even though the therapy is knocking her system down, she awoke from her nap amazingly bright eyed and smiling as she greeted me. With her there is always joy in the morning.

Thursday, March 7, 1996

It's seven am and I'm having a brief interlude of quiet and serenity. I hear the traffic outside the village. Many people out there are going to work, going to play. Here, time stands still. I know why they call it the Village. We are a community all on our own, with a different set of priorities. We come here to get our loved ones cured of a painful, frightening disease.

Here where it is the norm to see people bald, wearing a mask, tubes hanging out of blouses and shirts, wheel chairs, uniforms, lab coats, stethoscopes hanging around men's necks instead of ties. This is Amber's and my life for the next month and more.

Each day I feel more a part of this micro-community, where the conversations casually lean in the direction of before or after BMT, what type of cancer you or your loved one has, food that tastes like chemo, where to buy a soft hat for your hairless head to keep it warm and lots of knowledge and experience on how to get through this: One Day at a Time. This is our world, welcome to it.

Chapter Nine

Amber's ordeal

Sunday, March 10, 1996

I find it hard once again to motivate myself to write in my journal. My problem is I don't like to have to think about all of my newfound hardships. I completed radiation a few weeks ago and much has happened since then.

My throat became so painful I couldn't eat solids for about a week and I went through my eligibility tests (for the transplant) one after the other. In the middle of my 24-hour urine sample and just hours after my M.U.G.A. scan for my heart, I was called at 6:30 pm to head down to French Hospital to have my catheter placed. Dr. Howard, being as spur of the moment as he is, squeezed me in on a Friday night after a hellish week. I never got a break.

Coming home at around 11pm, me and my family arrived home to find my grandparents R.V. in the driveway. Surprise! One more stress to add to my list. Recovering from surgery was pretty hard. It didn't help being overwhelmed plus have my grandparents peeking in my room every now and then. Luckily they just stayed for the weekend and when they left I was relieved. It just takes too much to recuperate!

As things go I was told I had to go to City of Hope on Tuesday for a day of chemo to get my counts plunging and start my GCSF shots for ten days. (This is all part of the pre-transplant plan to kill the existing stem cells in the body and then boost the system with Neupogen to create more numerous strong ones.)

Once again I wasn't given much of a break. Everything is moving so fast, which I guess is good, but it's definitely difficult. I do better when I can deal with things one at a time. I haven't fully come to terms with this nuisance tube hanging out of me (the catheter called a double lumen Hickman) much less accepting this BMT. This is scary stuff. I have a lot of fear and anxiety that they haven't let me deal with. I want so much for this all to be over with and be successful at getting rid of this awful disease.

What keeps me hopeful is that little Elena is going through it, too and if a five-year-old has the guts then so can I. All I can do now is pray for strength and courage.

For Elena

I pray you Heavenly Father wait
To bring Elena to the gate
Her body frail and yet so strong
Her flesh of ivory
Her voice a song
She draws and paints
A child like few
With angels' breath
And hope anew
The road ahead
In faith must be
A stronger child
We'll never see
As sweet Elena
Heaven sent
A guiding star
God's will has meant

Janine
1/96

Chapter Ten

A tidal wave is predicted

Tuesday, March 12, 1996

Now that the two days of chemo are done, Amber's stem cell harvest will begin. I'm feeling a bit insecure and apprehensive about the tidal wave that's about to engulf us. The collection will take place at City of Hope and that will require trips there and lots of time surrounding the actual procedure. There is no way to know how long this process will take. It depends on her body's ability to grow new cells. In its weakened state, I am doubtful it will happen fast.

I must take this one moment at a time. So far I have mustered the strength and mastered my emotions surrounding giving her the shot each night. Her Dad holds her hand and I give the poke. We have a routine that involves putting Emla cream on the sight, hopefully dulling the pain involved with pushing the thick serum into her flesh. If I miss the spot we medicate it could mean unnecessary pain, so I have to be accurate. Having Tom here right now is such a relief. He takes some of the burden off my shoulders. We are both intent on saving her from any discomfort if at all possible.

Soon, we will be leaving our home and traveling down to the hospital to stay for the duration of the transplant. Our dear friends, Karen and Wes, have offered their motor home for me to live in while Amber is in the BMT ward. The village housing is only available while the patient is staying with the caregiver leading up to and recovering from the actual transplant. I will be able to park the motor home on the grounds within walking distance of the BMT ward. That way I can stay with her as long as possible each day in her hospital room, then walk "home" when she goes to sleep at night.

There is so much paperwork to do I am overwhelmed. Insurance forms, student loan deferments, SSI for Amber, correspondence to the University of San Diego to request she be allowed to attend again once this whole thing is over that includes her financial aid, and blah, blah, blah.

I am still trying to finish one class at a time that I took incompletes in at Cal Poly. My decision to do this is becoming less and less important to me. It was a former life I have no need for right now.

Thursday, March 14, 1996

The days are flying by now. So much to do, so little time to do it all. I want to keep up with Amber's Angels and give them a progress report. I also need to disinfect the house because Amber's white blood count is crashing and she is ripe for any bug that creeps into our house. Bridgett hasn't been much help lately. I guess she is rebelling again. Great timing. I pity the parents of adolescents. It is a thankless job for a long while. I had dreams of her last night as a baby, toddling along, sweet and smiling and soft. How I wish I could go back to those days.

Interlude

"High ho, high ho, it's off to lunch we go." My little ducklings trailing behind me, the lure of a Happy Meal keeping them in tow, "Let's go to the park and eat, Mommy." And why not? I had the pleasure of being home with my little girls and time was not an issue. "Shall we, girls," I opened the backdoor of our Chevy Caprice and they hopped into the back seat. "I need to hear the click, click of the seat belts before we can go. After all, you are the only Amber and Bridgett I have and I don't want anything bad to happen to either of you."

The park between Fourth and Second Street in the North Valley of Albuquerque, NM, featured a small playground, lots of grass, trees and a picnic table. Not unlike any other city park, this one was next to a McDonald's, and before they began putting playgrounds in the restaurants, mom's frequented this park with their toddlers.

"Let's eat first, then you can play." Amber was eyeballing the thing that goes round and round and would make any adult barf just looking at it. "Ok, Mommy." Her sissy followed her lead, and they both scrambled up to sit on the bench of the picnic table. Two bites later they were begging me to let them go play.

I watched as they began spinning round and round, my reflexes honed to jump to the rescue if needed. I winced as Amber drug her foot on the dirt. Those were $30 shoes. Oh well. So what if I paid more for their shoes than my own, their feet were growing and hopefully mine weren't.

"How about some ice cream?" My words weren't out of my mouth yet when they began to exit the spinning apparatus, not mindful of the motion they were engaged in and the lack of it they would step out on. Amber hit first, tumbling into the dirt. "Mommy!" Bridgett froze, still going around. Oh my God. I ran. Scooping her up in my arms, eyes still on Bridgett, I managed to stop the crazed monster and get her off. Amber was crying that hard cry any Mother's body tingles over. My mother-in-law called it the "ooh-who" feeling. A scrape, the kind that grates the skin raw instantly and burns like fire, was on both her knees. "I'm so sorry, honey," the guilt crashing down on me for not keeping her safe, "Let me kiss it and make it better."

An hour later, ice cream in hand, we sat very still on the same picnic bench. I vowed I would never let anything hurt my baby again.

Chapter Eleven

What do you do?

Saturday, March 16, 1996

    Alas, just as I had no control over the playground equipment of ten years ago, I have no control over what these complicated machines will do to my daughter's body in the present. None of this is entirely predictable, although there are some documented side effects that scare the crap out of me. I keep hoping she will be the one who avoids these, but there are just no guarantees.

    One of the results of high dose chemotherapy has been thrush, and Amber can hardly swallow. Because her white cell count is way down, her mouth is broken out in sores. She is listless and quite frail already and yet has so much more to go through. I don't know how much she can handle without giving up. The road ahead is really dangerous and as life threatening as the cancer itself.

    Her C.A.T. scan was done yesterday. With her counts so low, she had to wear a surgical mask while in the hospital. We saw her friend, Erin, who had just finished a bone scan. I'm not sure, but I think that suggests the pain she's been in may be due to the cancer spreading to her bones. My heart sank when I saw her in the wheel chair. While the girls talked, Robin and I did as well. As usual, waiting for these test results is a common thread between our families and having a scan on Friday means the weekend will be very long and apprehensive. The three W's,: Waiting, Wondering, Worrying.

We ended our day with a visit with Dr. Dan, who refers to the transplant as the "Amber Carter treatment." Even though he is not Amber's doctor officially, he is still watching out for her and prescribed some liquid Lortab to ease the pain in her throat so she can manage to eat some solid foods.

Sunday, March 17, 1996

I couldn't sleep past 6:30 this morning. I had Erin and her family on my mind. A phone call last evening to Robin was so therapeutic for me. We shared our thoughts and concerns for our daughters, and she even said preparing for the transplant makes their situation look not so bad. I don't envy them at this point either. What kind of treatment protocol will they put Erin on if the cancer has spread to her bones? This is nothing short of torture. There are so many questions and no answers. There are so many answers we don't want to hear. It is a Catch 22 at best.

Somehow we find our way through the struggle, but it's a real task to maintain any semblance of normality and sanity. Kind of like knowing there will be an earthquake, but you don't know where or how big it will be, so you finally give up on when the inevitable will happen and proceed with the mundane tasks every human does: Planning dinner, which for one of the family consists of liquids, or cleaning the house until your fingers bleed, or digging in the garden so no one will see your tears falling into the flowers. Or maybe you get on the computer and look up clinical trials, the latest on chemical therapies, statistics and percentages of survival for your child's type of cancer. And when you get there, you wish you hadn't. When all else fails you put on a movie and hope you can sit and zone out the truth for a couple of hours. You screen your phone calls because if one more person calls and says they are sorry, you think you will hammer the receiver into a million tiny pieces. And you pray…that's what you do.

Chapter Twelve

The natives are restless

Wednesday, March 20, 1996

We are back at City of Hope and as soon as I opened the door to our apartment, Bridgett paged me. When I called her the shit hit the fan.

"Why are you having Aunt Joan come here to baby-sit me? I am old enough to take care of myself. For your information I'm 16 and not a baby anymore. How embarrassing. And you didn't even tell me." She was crying and yelling. It was too much.

"She won't be your babysitter, she'll be your companion while I am here with Amber. I thought you would need someone to talk to since your Dad will be working nights." I was so exhausted from the three-hour drive and this topped it off.

"I don't want her to stay with me. I will be all right by myself."

"Let's not go into this right now. I am doing the best I can. I can't be in two places at once."

"Thanks a lot, Mom." She hung up. Then comes the guilt hammer to add to my discomfort.

Amber and I got settled in and got in bed. This was the longest day ever.

"Everything's going to be ok, Mommy," my little roomie assured me, "Bridgett just misses you, that's all. Goodnight. I love you mucho."

"Goodnight my sweetie. I love you more."
Sleep came finally, fitfully.

Thursday, March 20, 1996

Today we bounced around the corridors of the hospital all day long. Sometime during our lunch in the cafeteria, Amber broke down. The meetings with the nutrition-ist, home health care nurse, and having her blood drawn, followed by a visit with Dr. Spyberg, took their toll. She was hungry, angry, lonely, and tired. No amount of ration-alizing would comfort her. Serenity was out of the question. In a corner, by the soda machine, she let it all out. I was there and so was God, and as I received my comfort, I passed it onto her by validating her feelings. I admitted I felt overwhelmed, too. We finally ate and reported to ambulatory where she would be receiving a platelet transfu-sion from some kind donor. When we arrived there was laying room only. I pulled up a doctor's swivel stool and sat down next to her bed. I had brought a portable Backgammon game with me and once the nurse plugged Amber in we played a few games. It took four hours of drip, drip, drip, and finally she got released to go back to our apartment where we watched some television and fell into bed. It had been some day. No news from home. My guess was that Bridgett got her anger out on me and was probably giving her Dad the quiet treatment. Whatever was happening there would have to take care of itself. I had my own hands full here putting out my own fires. I was forcing myself to stay in this place and time. I had no room or strength left to do otherwise.

Chapter Thirteen

In God's time

Friday, March 22, 1996

I got back from City of Hope tonight after another hectic week. This was stem cell collection week, which began with a rocky start. My (blood) counts were too low as a result of the chemo and radiation so it was postponed until Wednesday and after a platelet transfusion the day before. Stem cell collection is pretty harmless. My only complaint is that it lasts too long. Four hours is a long time to be sitting in one position. Luckily they have movies to watch and my own personal TV with earphones.

Anyway my collection is happening pretty slow. (Goal is 2.0, after two days I have .24) so it looks like everything is going to be put off another week. (Not that I'm excited about TBI (total body irradiation) or anything!) I just pray that next week we're more successful, because I'm sick of these GCSF (Neupogin) shots everyday.

I'm starting to loose my hair again. Tonight it was coming out in chunks and I have a bald spot on the side of my head. I swear this is one of the hardest parts, so I've decided that tomorrow I'm going to have my Dad buzz it off before it really starts falling. Somehow it makes me feel better to have control over the situation. I'm deciding when I want it all to come off instead of being tortured for a week or so feeling helpless. I know it's coming out regardless. I'm just getting it over with so I won't be depressed each day a little more falls out!

Chapter Fourteen

<u>Motherhood is insanity</u>

Tuesday, March 26, 1996

The weekend was short and emotional. Tom got a lesson in snooping through his daughter's things. He said he wasn't looking for anything, it just popped up at him. A note he found in Bridgett's dance bag made a huge impact on their relationship. Lessons were learned here and the teacher was Fate. I was the unfortunate one caught in the middle.

Tom had called me the afternoon we were coming home from the hospital and was strangely quiet. I could tell he had something to tell me, but I was not prepared for this. He had "found" a note written to Bridgett that inferred she was pregnant. What? My heart and stomach collided; my head was spinning out of control. Here I was with our oldest daughter being prepped for a major life-threatening procedure and he was laying this on me by telephone.

Now there is always the knowledge this kind of thing can happen, and with all the time I had been away and her not having me to talk to had me thinking. When she was crying about Aunt Joan coming to stay with her, was there another reason for her tears? My mind was going crazy with what ifs. I always blamed myself for any wrong-doing my children may have stepped into. Why is that? Is it a mother's nature? As if being guilty was easier to handle than raising a child to be so. To be guilty is part of the code and it was easier to blame myself than the innocent child I gave birth to.

Because I was away taking care of my other daughter who had cancer, it was my fault Bridgett might be pregnant. And why did Amber have this dreaded disease anyway? I even thought somehow making Amber's baby food must have been why, or the move we made out here to California had to have a serious effect on her system to make her more susceptible to it. Hell, if I'd only put her in a plastic bubble from birth, maybe that would have done the trick. Make that two bubbles.

So on and on I condemned myself for being a terrible mother. If only I had… maybe if I…I should have. This kind of thinking can make a person insane. I call it my own version of the Domino Effect. Each thought would build and fall on top of the next more awful one, until I would find my heart beating wildly, my lungs breathing rapidly, and that I had driven 400 miles and didn't know how I got there.

By the time I got home, I had accused myself of sleeping with a boy, getting pregnant and, through mystical osmosis had transferred this condition to my unsuspecting 17-year-old virgin daughter. I walked in the door apologizing profusely for being a negligent mother out on the town. I told you motherhood would make you insane.

In a moment of clarity, my husband informed me the rumor he had delivered a la telephone was unfounded and Bridgett piped in, "If you hadn't read my private notes you wouldn't have been so worried." So there…

Chapter Fifteen

<u>Motor home, away from home, going home</u>

Wednesday, March 27, 1996

     We spent the remainder of the "lost weekend" preparing for going down to the hospital with our borrowed motor home. Wes kindly gave Tom a training session on driving the 27-foot casa and it was carefully parked in our driveway for the trip down on Friday. My sister, Joan, is scheduled to fly to Pasadena on Saturday, then drive to the hospital in Duarte and pick up Tom and Bridgett. They will be bringing the motor home down for me to stay in for the duration of Amber's transplant procedure.

     The TBI has been postponed for a week due to Amber's slow stem cell collection. She was uptight yesterday about the possibility of her doctor forcing solutions and doing the cell collection and the TBI in the same week. After voicing her displeasure, they decided to wait until April 6th to be admitted into the hospital. Until then, we will remain tenants of the village and she will be shuttled to her appointments from there.

Tuesday, March 26, 1996

     Yesterday I donated platelets at the donor center where they separate blood components into platelets and red cells, and also where the stem cell collection takes place. I knew Amber would be needing platelets soon, and since I have the same blood type, I tried to make sure the bank had some of mine. I could designate them especially for her, but if she didn't need them within the allotted expiration period, they would be thrown away. As it turned out, she didn't get mine this time, but some other needy patient did. Isn't that how it should work? The haves give to the have-nots.

The miracle of transfusions for people is worth the effort. If it weren't for those volunteers with Amber's blood type, she would die from the chemotherapy treatments that kill off cancer cells and blood cells. The donor's procedure is not without its discomfort. To give platelets, two I.V. needles are needed, one for removing the whole blood and another in the other arm to send the blood into the aphaeresis machine that separates platelets from red cells. Then they are bagged separately for the patients that need them.

Being able to give my blood to my precious Amber meant I could finally do something more than just care for her.

Thursday, March 28, 1996

I'm here in the apartment alone. Amber is at the aphaeresis center getting her stem cells collected. I counted 22 shots of GCSF so far that I have had to stick her with. In addition to that she has her blood drawn weekly, has received three blood transfusions, and seven collections of stem cells. Her body is a walking pincushion.

Karen, our nurse coordinator, says if enough stem cells aren't collected soon, Amber may have to have a bone marrow extraction. Hearing this put Amber over the edge. She still thinks she must be doing something wrong. She is trying so hard to keep up her faith, but this wasn't what she wanted to hear. I had to jump in as cheerleader and give her a pep talk. I let her cry and she lost hope for a short while. It's hard to imagine how frustrating and helpless she must feel. I just try to comfort her, give her empathy, try not to fix, and somehow bring out the positive from all of this. Sometimes it's damn near impossible.

I keep saying, "In God's time, a day at a time," and I must believe it. So far I'm in today and don't want to think about next week. I just want to be home for a couple of days to hug my husband, Bridgett, and pet the cat.

Chapter Sixteen

What if she were your daughter?

Tuesday, April 2, 1996

We were sitting in the lobby of the hospital. It was ten o'clock at night. This area in daytime was a zoo of people and activity. Now it was ghostly and quiet to the point of being eerie. The entire day was crashing down on me and Amber. At last she could put the difficult day behind her. Earlier in the day, while we were in the cafeteria, somewhere between the pizza and tuna melts, she had another meltdown. I tried to comfort her and brought her to the edge of the room. It was all becoming so overwhelming. She let the tears flow. I wondered just how much she could take.

Our visit with Dr. Spyberg first thing in the morning ended up being his au revoir, or should I say adios. He was going on vacation to Venezuela for two weeks. Great. So much for building a bond with her doctor. In one week she would be receiving her transplant and he wouldn't even be here to see her through it. I was pissed. She was hurt.

Amber was being assigned to Dr. Sapuir, a pediatric BMT doctor. Our next meeting was with her. She was a compassionate, quiet doctor with a nice bedside manner. At least we approved of the pinch hitter. Still, it was so weird to have this happen at such a late date, and right before the big transplant day.

Stem cell collection took place after our meeting with the new doc, followed by a blood draw for pre-BMT testing. The lab technician took 13 vials of blood, and afterward Amber needed a transfusion. No wonder, they had just drained it all out of her. Off we went to ambulatory where she began to receive red blood cells, and potassium.

While Amber was receiving her transfusion, I went back to the apartment to get a sweater. On the table in the dining area was a box filled with prescription drugs, bags of saline, syringes, tubing, and standing there was an I.V. pole. Whoever left it there must have heard my meager brain on overload because the phone rang at that moment and the person began a litany of instructions that I only heard half of. I was totally on over load. Just buying her the low-bacteria food the day before along with rules about wiping anything she put her mouth on with alcohol had me spinning. Now I was expected to be her nurse.

I hung up the phone and decided to call our nurse, Karen. It was four days before Amber's scheduled admittance to the hospital, but I could see it would be four damn long days at this rate. I walked back to the hospital and sat with Amber while she received her transfusion. Meanwhile I put a call into Karen and asked her to meet us in the lobby. By the time she got there, Amber was a zombie and I must have looked how I felt. Bedraggled, angry, and tired. I began to tell her about our day.

"And here it is, ten o'clock and Amber has not had one moments rest, other than receiving the transfusion." I couldn't hide my anger and had to hold myself back from crying. "Now I'm expected to go back to our apartment and learn how to be her nurse. Look at her." Amber had fallen asleep on the couch next to me.

"I can see your point. Your insurance company is setting the rules here. I'll do what I can." She was listening.

It all became clear to me. The stupid insurance people were trying to save money by having me be her nurse instead of forking over the money to admit her into the hospital. I was furious.

"Let me ask you this, Karen. Do you have any children?"

"Yes, I do," she hesitated, " I have a daughter the same age as Amber."

"If this was your daughter, what would you do?"

She looked into my eyes deeply, picked up her cell phone and dialed the bone marrow unit.

"Would you get a room ready for Amber Carter immediately."

Bingo.

Chapter Seventeen

The Garden of Gethsemane

Tuessday, April 2, 1996

    Once Amber was situated in her room in the unit, I went to the apartment by myself. This was definitely the most alone I had ever been. You could say Amber and I had been joined at the hip, and now we were surgically separated. She was nestled into her 10 X 10 foot hospital room, and I was a block away in the village. It felt like a mile away to me. Hadn't we just had a victory? Then why did I feel so defeated and sad?

    I should have been able to fall into bed and crash, but instead I had the most cleansing cry ever. I cried for everything: the sweater I had lost the day before with the Angel wings on it, the idiot doctor on his way to Venezuela, my home, my Bridgett, my husband, my own bed. I cried right down to the bare bones, to the tips of my toes and back up again. Somewhere along the road to loneliness, I fell asleep.

Wednesday, April 3, 1996

    Today is Amber's first TBI session, that's an acronym for total body radiation. She is so scared of this. I'm not sure why, except she's never had it before and the unknown is always scary. I went to the lobby in the unit to get a snack. At the table was seated a young woman dressed in a hospital gown. I introduced myself. Her name was Michaela and she was post BMT and about to be released to the village where her subsequent recovery would take place. She was all alone. Her husband had divorced her, and her children were with him. How sad, I thought. Here she was fighting for her life and no one was here to help her. I told her how Amber was feeling about this next radiation. She insisted on following me back to talk to her about it.

There was more than just the common ground of cancer treatments between the two women. They chatted about attending Allan Hancock College, and that this was just a bump in the road off the course of education. As I listened, Michaela explained to Amber what to expect. She said the techs were very kind and considerate, and would stop at any time if she just nodded to them. Having an experienced human being take the time to talk to her made all the difference to Amber. Armed with the knowledge of what was about to happen, she awaited the attendant to wheel her to the next battleground and the hidden arsenal in the bowels of the hospital.

The picture of my sweet daughter haunts me as I write. I can see her inside the radiation room, standing against the wall harnessed to this contraption, hands gripping handles, her childlike innocence contrasting the brutality of the latest array of tortures. Her precious baldhead was pressing against the wall as if she were trying desperately to back away. I will never forget this image as long as I live.

Each moment in this chamber is an eternity for her. As I watch her from the monitor, I stand alongside the technician who I must remind myself is on Amber's side, trying to help her win the war, while my daughter struggles to stand up and receive the radiation. Only two minutes pass and she needs a break. I rush in with the techs permission and try to soothe her in any way I can. She feels so weak, she says, like she's about to faint. Indeed.

After many starts and stops, her first full body radiation experience is over. The ride back to her room in the wheel chair is much welcomed. I tag along behind with my heart in my throat. I must not let her see me cry, but it is difficult holding back my tears when I see her weakly smiling and being courteous to the attendant even after what she has just been through.

By 9:00 am, Amber finally asks the nurse for some Compazine, an anti-emetic. Knowing it would make her sleepy, she held off as long as possible so she could stay awake with me. The sight and smell of food makes her throw up. Soon, they will be putting her on an I.V. of liquid supplement they call TPN. It is standard for all patients in this unit. Food is not a friend. She has not been able to keep down much. Her weight is at 112 lbs.

It is hard to believe this time last month we were attending Weight Watcher meetings. At least that was a fulfilling time for her. She reached her goal weight, grew out her hair enough to have it styled by our friend, Becka, and could fit into her precancer jeans. I must remember her that way to get me through these next few weeks. After today I know how the slippery slope will be on the uphill climb towards her transplant date. Thank God she is in the hospital now under constant watch by the nurses used to this kind of thing. I can't imagine me trying to care for her by myself. Just getting her to and from the hospital on the shuttle they provided was becoming impossible.

After Amber went to sleep, I walked outside and ate my lunch in the rose garden. It was peaceful and I was able to let myself rest. Later on in the afternoon I brought Amber back with me and as I pushed her wheel chair, she felt good enough to enjoy the beautiful roses and the kids playing in the yard of the children's hospital. They were having an Easter egg hunt in the park and some of the siblings had been invited to visit and participate. It was fun to watch. We took pleasure in the little things we used to take for granted. I couldn't help but think this was like Jesus walking in the garden before he went through his final ordeal. Soon Amber would be put through more suffering and it was beginning to register just how much.

Back inside her room, I watched her sleeping. It's such a lonely time for me. I'm sad to think of our family being split apart. Bridgett doesn't get to see her dad because he's on the night shift, and I am 200 miles away. She must feel like an orphan, poor thing. At least I know Joan is there for a companion. She is truly one of Amber's Angels.

Chapter Eighteen

<u>Spending time together, and apart</u>

Saturday, April 6, 1996

    Amber's more than halfway through radiation treatments. She is on a mostly liquid diet now, barely able to keep broth and soda crackers down. She still manages a smile to everyone around her. We are both looking forward to seeing her dad, sister, and Aunt Joan this weekend. Tomorrow they will be here. She is slightly anxious because the next round of chemo starts then and she doesn't want them to see her sick. She is so considerate and worries too much about others. Anyway, we are both excited for our family to come and visit. By this time tomorrow night we will all be together.

Saturday, April 7, 1996

    Well, the other half of our family is here and I feel complete! I've missed Bridgett a lot more than I thought. She and I haven't been close since she started puberty, but she's coming out of it finally and for all those times I wanted to kill her, I take them back now.

    So, let's not dwell on missing stuff. I'm so grateful they came down. It's very lonely for me here.

    Amber began chemo today. VP16 flowed into her veins for four hours. She is wiped out. Her body is purging liquid and solid waste constantly. The Lasix is responsible for part of that. Bridgett is keeping her company while Tom and I move our stuff from the village apartment to the motor home. It will be slightly closer to the hospital where I spend most of my time.

While we were moving, Joan went to donate platelets. It is a sacrifice we all feel motivated to do. There is little else that can be done to physically help Amber aside from giving her our prayers. There is an element of suffering involved that makes it come from the heart, literally pumping part of us into a bag in hopes she will receive it. At the very least, the bank is being kept full for other patients in need like Amber. Her Dad proudly came back after his donation and said they called him the "platelet factory." He was grinning from ear to ear as though he had run a big race and came in first. And so he has won the satisfaction of giving some of himself for his daughter.

Bridgett wanted to help by giving as well, but at 110 lbs it was not advisable. She wants to help her sissy out, but that is a risk for her own health and I know it has done Amber a lot of good just seeing her. She thoughtfully brought her an Easter basket and plush rabbit on her own. I see her becoming a mature young lady.

After the family went to the motor home to sleep, I stayed with Amber and decided to spend the night with her. She is now purging at both ends and all at once. The poor little thing—she is so helpless right now. I keep reminding her (and myself) that this is the path for cure. The infantry is going in to clean out the enemy. There are casualties along the way, the other body functions revolting from the skirmish. Well, the good guys are going to win—that's all there is to it !

I am feeling like I'm trying to catch a cold. Oh, I can't get sick now. I won't. I'm wearing a surgical mask just in case. Amber's WBC is at 1.1—she's ripe for infection

Monday, April 8, 1996

It's 10:00 am and the nurse just started Amber's Cytoxin drip. This is her last dose of chemo and she warned us that Amber may vomit etc. following the two hours it is administered. She is trying to sleep, but fluids running through her to keep her hydrated and to prevent the chemo from sitting in her bladder and kidneys make her go pee every ten minutes or so. You'd think they would just put a catheter in, but instead she has to get up and down to the porta-potty seated next to her bed.

Her platelets are holding steady at 110 and WBC is 1.6, with hemoglobin at 8.8. Things are looking stable for now. This is the calm before the storm.

Every evening after shift changes, I talk to the night shift nurse and size her up. If I like her manners, I feel comfortable leaving. If not, I stick around as late as possible. Last night she was a nice one, could speak English well, (some of them don't) and had a good bedside manner. I felt ok to leave her and sleep in the motor home. The night before I stayed with her and didn't sleep very well in the foldout recliner chair. I hate to leave, but if I don't get my rest, I'll get sick and be no good to her.

It was lonely after I left Amber. The new accommodations, the late hour, the dark, all made for a scary setting. Even though the RV is closer, the new surroundings made me uneasy. Also, I had been with my family all day yesterday, in and out, a flurry of activity. Now it was all too quiet and smelled funny, the smell of nobody, of loneliness. I watched some TV, cleaned out my purse, cried, changed into my jammies and tried to comfort myself. When I turned off the television, it was another adjustment to the quiet and darkness.

I began thinking. Why was this happening to us? We are a good family, trying to straighten our lives out and just be happy and then this just slams us all down. And why Amber? I just don't get it. After this short bout of self-pity, I settled down with my rosary beads and mouthed each prayer trying to believe their meaning. I finally just gave up and fell asleep.

Chapter Nineteen

<u>Somewhere out there</u>

Monday, April 8, 1996

 The chemo is really cooking inside Amber's body. She has been vomiting and had diarrhea since early this morning when I got to her room. It's now 10:30 pm and there can't be anything left in this poor child's body. She hasn't eaten solid food that has stayed down since Saturday. It's so hard to watch her puke and puke with nothing there but spit. She is so weak and miserable. It was hard to help her today, not because of the mess, just because I can't help her feel better no matter what I try. She didn't even want a foot rub. I don't want her to give up.

 We had a spiritual moment together today that helped. Father Ron from our church back home had given me a special container to hold communion wafers. When Amber was too sick to attend mass, I would receive my own and ask for one to be placed in it for her. I carried this with me on our last trip here. Today Amber and I gave each other communion and prayed together before she got so sick. It was really cleansing and hopeful.

 I pray that she will be able to sleep through the night. When I left her she was finally dozing. I gently kissed her balding head and softly walked out of her room. My short journey to the motor home was dark and foreboding. It seemed like I was carrying the load of two people on my shoulders. Indeed, I was.

As I climbed up into my temporary home, I couldn't help but feel that longing again for my own 200 miles away. I looked up into the black sky and saw the same stars that shown above my little house in Grover Beach. There has always been some comfort in knowing this is shared with my loved ones while we are separated. When we moved to California, my mom would remind me of Feival, the little mouse that sang *Somewhere Out There* in the movie *American Tale*, and I would cherish the words and think of my family back in New Mexico, especially her. Now, I was thinking of my babies. One in the hospital, and one back home. My heart ached to have them beside me.

This is only the beginning of the long journey of Amber's cure from cancer. God continues to provide me with the strength to help her go on. I wish he could also provide me with some sense of it all. Her pain is my pain, what mother does not wish that away? This child of mine, her future, lies in the hands of doctors and nurses. Do they realize what a precious package they hold there? I am adamant they do. It is all I can do aside from prayer right now. To remind them she is my present given to me on the day of her birth and I am not ready for her to be taken away. My deepest fears crowd into my brain in the dark of night and loneliness. Here, I can write my helpless words onto innocent paper. My pen is poised and ready to glean my sorrow from my fingertips that are an extension of my body. It's as if they have their own power to pull the ache I feel in my heart, through my blood that turns into ink to be words writing the horrible truth. I am afraid my child may die.

Chapter Twenty

<u>Transplant Day</u>

Wednesday, April 10, 1996

The day is finally here. I went out and bought balloons to commemorate Amber's "second birthday." As they float around her head, she sheepishly grins at her incorrigible Mom. She's so sick she doesn't have the energy to be embarrassed so she just grins and bears it.

It's ten o'clock and she is receiving her fifth bag of stem cells. They have been cryogenically preserved, and they are icy cold, so cold we keep piling blankets on top of her to try and keep her warm, beginning with her favorite afghan, and ending with the kitty quilt grandma Verna made special for this event, and three other blankets in between. She peeks out from under the mound with her little skullcap on her head and looks like the proverbial "bug in a rug."

Each bag of cells has to be checked by the first nurse, read off to another, before the third nurse can administer them. Once they were harvested from Amber, they were radiated, frozen, and put into storage for this day. Funny how the transport container is nothing more than a large red igloo cooler that could be some construction workers lunch.

I stand in amazement and watch the bags pass from one nurses hand to another like a runner's baton, careful not to drop, checking each one for authenticity, quickly hooking each one up to drip into the tubing attached to Amber's I.V. With the help of the lymph nodes that have been poisoned and irradiated, the re-introduced, radiated cells will now flow into her body and will be transported throughout with the hope of eventual homeostasis.

There is no fanfare, honking horns, no confetti, only three nurses working feverishly to transfuse these cells within the allotted time. The recipient is trying her best to withstand the enormously cold cells entering her body creating stomach cramping, headache, diarrhea, and irregular blood pressure. The physical ramifications are not fully realized by the lay person, but the medical personnel know full well the impact on the body from this abusive attempt to annihilate the cancer.

I feel distanced from this action, helpless to a fault, as if I am watching a movie. I want to close my eyes at the bad parts, but am glued to the spot not able to move or blink away the terror I'm feeling.

Amber is mainly uncomfortable, irritated, antsy, and very, very cold. She wears an unusual frown on her brow, eyes of steel, painfully holding on minute by minute. I stand aside, unable to fathom what she is going through. I just kept thinking this was another first for my baby along with the memory of her first steps, first day at school, first kiss, and now, first transplant. The tears come and rest in my heart.

Amber coughs a little and finally settles down for sleep. I take a deep breath. The machines are making their bumping sound, pumping the required medications into her port of entry giving immediate relief finally. I stand and watch her sleep.

I hear the sounds of nurses and patients in the hall, someone's little child running and laughing, just another day for most, but not for me. This is the first day of the cure for Amber and the first day of her new cancer-free life. From here the only way is up. Like a bird that's been caged, she will be set free. It's a long road to get there and the journey is beginning today.

I'm grateful I can be here with her on this day as I was on the day of her birth. She is reborn today. I am here to witness this moment and I relish in it.

Chapter Twenty-one

No pain, no gain?

Friday, April 12, 1996

    Amber's fever is at 102, she has major throat pain, and she is still vomiting this awful thick, green stuff. She is just plain miserable! Hard to believe just a week ago she could meet her dad and sissy at the village. So much has happened since their visit. Her spirit is still pretty good but she feels crappy. Morphine is being pushed every two hours now and Dr. Sapuir has ordered a drip so it will be continuous beginning this afternoon. They say Amber is on track for her symptoms and discomfort. This is hard for me to watch. She holds onto her partner (the I.V. pole on rollers) with the beeping machines pumping her medications (there are six different ones.) I make sure none of the tubes get caught or run over. It's a major ordeal just to get her to the restroom that is three feet away. I feel so helpless when all I can do is hold her puke pan, sit by her side and try to comfort her.

Saturday, April 13, 1996

    I'm sitting in the rose garden and it's a beautiful sunny day. The scent of the flowers is drifting around me and giving me some peace of mind. I can hear the little waterfall trickling behind me, and the birds are chirping away. In the distant background is the ever-present sound of traffic on the freeway and people going lots of places all around me. My world is small and quite predictable. No surprises here, only the continued hope of recovery for Amber. I wish I could trade some of her pain for this serenity I'm feeling right now.

Meanwhile, she is getting my platelets today. That makes me feel really good. I knew eventually she would have my blood swimming in her body. What a wonderful feeling. It is the ultimate and only gift I can give her that comes close to what I wish I could do. I wish I could trade places with her altogether.

Once my visit to the garden is over, I will go back to the hospital, wash my hands, don my face mask and surgical gown and be with Amber the rest of the day. Because her white cells are so low, the risk for infection is great. Anyone who visits her has to be covered. They place a mask over the door of her hospital room to signify that fact when her WBC is less than 100.

Amber has been pretty drugged up these days so our communication is limited. I have been calling home a lot and my conversations with Tom are a nice distraction. I also get a chance to talk with other caregivers occasionally when I go and do laundry in the village, but they are strictly superficial. No deep feelings are shared, or tears shed, just the realities of our separate situations as we are bonded together by our circumstances. I wish there was a meeting for us like they had at the Wellness Community in Pasadena. There, we could share our deepest thoughts and fears and receive validation. Here we are all just strangers in a strange land.

Amber has been in the hospital for 13 days so far and it looks like she'll be here for probably 13 more.

Monday, April 22, 1996

So many people come to mind as I ponder the last three weeks. We have been meeting patients on the BMT Unit and their families that are going through what we are. Right next door is a man who plays for the Mighty Ducks, and his wife is pregnant. They are from Czechoslovakia and have been here four months. She sleeps in his room every night. Then there is Chris who had two types of leukemia at the same time. His wife Cilda and their three-year-old daughter, Sara, have been here at least half a year. Roy has been in isolation so we have never met him, but his son, James, visits with me in the lounge sometimes. All of us wishing each other well, concerned with progress of our loved ones. Words aren't always necessary, a look, a smile, a wringing of the hands, all of us as positive as we can be for each other. We are in our own micro community.

My friend, Donna, came to visit us. She was a sight for sore eyes. It feels like we've been here an eternity, and when someone comes in from the "outside" it is such a pleasure. Tommy's friend, Mark came all the way down here from our hometown just to give blood for Amber. That meant an entire day of driving. What a guy. Of course our own Dad came to visit us a few days after and that was exciting. It is very hard for him to get away, but he managed to do so and it perked Amber right up. Her white blood cells were up so no mask was needed and her daddy could see her smile. We managed an hour or two alone and he caught me up on home news. Things seem to be going ok, no trauma dramas to report. I had a deep, cleansing cry on his shoulder that was completely spontaneous, but much needed. I guess I don't realize how much I am holding in.

9:00 P.M.

Roy passed away tonight. This man didn't know us, or we him, but his son had become close to me. James is Amber's age and now is without a father. It's so hard to watch such a struggle for life when at the same time death is around for any one of us. I laid in bed with Amber for a while and felt her tears upon my face. The feeling of having someone die in a room next to us was so seriously sacred and it put a different sort of importance on our own fragile situation. As a mother, I dared not imagine for a second what that must have felt like for James. I did not ever want to know.

REFLECTION `96

College days interrupted
Instead of a dorm room
you got room 722
equipped with a porta potty and I V stand
No roommate to talk to
instead, a full time nurse and mom

I wanted to buy you a throw rug
to step out on
so your feet wouldn't touch the cold floor
something blue and fluffy
to decorate your room, nice and cozy
But, the wheels wouldn't roll over it
so, that was out

Let's do lunch!
Ok—what flavor glucose?
We have an array of barf pans

All color coordinated in drab yellow
All within easy reach
(You never know)

While your friends were making decisions
like—what should I wear to the frat party?
You were struggling to sit up or
make it around the corridor more than once
And "What shall I do with my hair?"
turned into, "I wish it would all fall out at once—-I hate the Mohawk look!"

While they listened to alternative
you were stuck in a time warp
of golden oldies
because mom was your friend and companion
So you put up with
"Don't leave me home-girl"
one more time
and giggled at her singing it

When your friends called
with their lame crises of mid-terms
you witnessed a person
dying in the room down the hall
and cried for someone you never met, yet knew so well

It's all part of your general ed.
Cancer 101, BMT 211, Recovery 310
Your professors have titles
Oncologist, hematologist, radiologist
The real teacher
is yourself
And you've earned an A plus
Congratulations on graduating

Janine
5/96 reflections of April BMT

Chapter Twenty-two

<u>Ache with nostalgia</u>

Sunday, April 28, 1996

As much as I wanted to keep up on writing through my BMT it was to say the least, impossible! Today is day +18 since my transplant. My second birthday is now April 10. TBI was as bad as I had expected and the mouth sores and sore throat were horrible. I was on morphine through most of my days so, to my gain, I don't remember every moment of pain. I am now in my third day in the village. It still isn't easy. I'm on TPN at night and during the day I try to force myself to eat. My Mom has been the best. She puts up with my morphine withdrawal mood swings and my on-going boughts of throwing up. I never expected that eating would be such a problem after my BMT, but is <u>so</u> hard. Nothing tastes good and often it won't stay down. Today I had my first pancakes. The first one came up, but being determined as I was I sat back down and tried it again. This one stayed down!

The reason I want to start eating so bad is because this is my only way to get home. The doctor won't release me until I can nourish myself without night time (TPN) nourishment. The past few days have been emotionally hard for me. First of all I can't stop worrying that my cancer isn't gone. Sometimes I feel mild pain in my neck and I think I feel a small bump. My worst fear is that this, too, hasn't worked. This is something I <u>really</u> need to work on or else I may sabotage all the work I've put into getting rid of this thing. So I'm writing positive affir-

mations to myself and trying hard not to think those awful thoughts.

"I am perfectly happy to be me. I am good enough just as I am. I love and approve of myself. I am joy expressing and receiving."

I'm listening to this song "Everybody Hurts" by REM, and the lyrics really pertain to me. The words speak of not giving up and hanging on. I think that it is a sign telling me that one day things will get better as long as I don't give up. It's the second time I've heard this song this week. Maybe it's coincidence, but I'd like to think God is somehow speaking to me the encouraging words I so desperately need.

Tuesday, April 29, 1996

I went to the doctor today and with much dread because I wanted to ask him if I could go home next weekend for Bridgett's confirmation. I worried all night "what if he says no" and worked myself up again. Seeing Bridge on her special day was so important to me I couldn't bear an answer of no. well with needless worries he told me I could go home for the weekend. I will have to come back on Monday or Tuesday and if I'm eating and doing good I can go home for good with the exception of check-ups. I was so relieved and mad that I had worried for no reason. I need to stop doing that. It just ends up making me unhappy and miserable. It's so hard to train yourself to have faith once you slip from remission. I find myself remembering when Dr.Dan told me that I was done with chemo. How I cried because I was so happy and then within a month it came back. I was so devastated and I never want that to happen again, but who can predict the future. Only God, and he has some sort of plan for me. I have to keep reminding myself of that. "Thy will be done."

Wednesday, May 1st

Today I woke up feeling a little less anxious and I got through the night without worrying about relapse. So I guess I've improved a little bit. My neck still seems to hurt mildly and I have a hard time distinguishing whether or not it is my neck. Sometimes I think I'm going crazy. The cause is most likely my sleeping positions which have had to be altered due to my Hickman (port) and my nighttime IV, but it's hard to convince myself of this. There's no way that my cancer could come back this quick after TBI and intense chemo, especially to the point of pain.

My Mom wants me to talk to my social worker, but I'm so stubborn I don't know how she could help me. I won't be happy until my first C.A.T. scan, which happens in the upcoming week or so, which I'm sure will say good news. (See how I'm trying to be positive!) Until then I need to stop worrying what if… It takes so much energy and precious time. So I'm praying dearly for strength to push these negative thoughts away, especially for this weekend at home. I don't want these worries to ruin it for me. As my Mom reminds me—Today is a present and here is where I need to be. Who knows what will happen tomorrow.

Chapter Twenty-three

<u>Seeds of doubt</u>

Thursday, May 2, 1996

    I went to the social worker today to talk about all of the feelings I've been having lately. It helped somewhat, but I continue to have sensations of tensions or mild pain in my neck and no matter what, I think about it. I am alerted to that area. The doctor said it felt the same today, as on Monday, which means it hasn't grown, so logically I couldn't be having pain there. My only explanation is that my bed here is so hard that it is irritating my neck and shoulder, but I can't help but wonder if it's back. My C.A.T. scan won't be for another week and we won't know anything until then. So finally this afternoon I couldn't stand thinking about it anymore and I took a pain pill. Not that I'm in total pain, I just wanted to stop focusing all of my thoughts to that area. I saw the pills and immediately thought ESCAPE! I know it was horrible, but at least for 3 or 4 hours I'll mellow out and enjoy the life I have right now. Obviously my Mom didn't know, but she would just worry about me.

    I'm going home tonight so I hope that being away (from this place) will make a difference. My biggest hope is the sensation will fade so I can focus my thoughts somewhere else. I'm sick of wondering if my biggest fear will come true. If it is back does that mean that there's nothing else they will do for me. Am I going to die at age 19 before my life ever really began? There are so many things I want to do and experience, like college, relationships, love and nor-

mality. This is what I mean by getting worked up, but I had to get these fears down and out of my thoughts. They are horrible thoughts.

I just pray that my nightmare will end and my life will begin. This is my only prayer…Life!

Power of love

"Do you believe, "
I said
"in the power of love?"
"Yes," she cried
and that above
all else seemed
right
and helped me through
the darkest night
My purpose clear
at last I see
to give my love
and to
receive
it back tenfold
then ten times ten
I'll not go through
these doubts again
but hold her close
and hold her
tight
and tell her love
will make it right
and we won't give up
without a
fight !

Janine

Chapter Twenty-four

<u>Home at last</u>

Thursday, May 2, 1996

Dr. Spyberg gave Amber permission to go home for the weekend even though she is still so very weak and on the liquid TPN for nourishment. We have to bring home Eddie (her I.V, pole and pump), but being there in our home, able to sleep in our own beds will be a treat. I see some cheerfulness returning at last. I hear hope in her voice that hasn't been there since this whole thing began. Bridgett's confirmation is on Sunday.

Monday, May 6, 1996

The sun is shining, the birds are singing, I am home. We had a busy weekend and now it's time to go back to the hospital and see if her doc will make this permanent and release her to Dr. Dan for continued care.

Tom, Amber and I had a great time watching Bridgett dance in a performance at the high school on Friday. "Kaleidoscope" is an annual fundraiser for the P.E. department that Amber and she have been in together in the past. Now it is Bridgett's turn to shine solo. Her confidence in her dancing really showed and I could tell she was happy we were there, and so were we!

On Sunday we attended her Holy Confirmation. She looked so grown up and got the recognition she deserved for all her hard work in preparation. Dr. Dan and his wife Mary Ellen were present as well as our good friends Karen and Wes and family. Afterwards we had a reception at our house. It was a fitting end to such a special week for her. The spotlight was on Bridgett for once. It felt good to do something for her for a change. She is growing up to be quite a mature and caring young lady. I have missed her tremendously.

Now we will have to make one last trek to City of Hope to have Dr. Spyberg read the latest C.A.T. scan done here. Taking the pictures to him will expedite the process.

Tuesday, May 7, 1996

Dr. Spyberg said Amber's C.A.T. scan and blood work looked very good, and that news was like finding a pearl in an oyster. As he was making his exit he called in his physicians assistant and ordered her to remove the Hickman line from Amber's breast. What? With just lidocaine injected to numb the immediate area she began to pull on the central line that had been surgically placed two months previous. This was really painful. As Amber held onto my hand, she was told to lie still. Scar tissue had formed around the cuff under her skin and the assistant kept working it around to get it lose. This procedure was done as an afterthought with not so much as a nod of the head. The tears were rolling down Amber's head, onto her ears, dangling off her earrings. What a pitiful sight…more pain, more torture. Finally, mercifully, the cuff tore away and she wrapped the tubing around her finger and slowly pulled it out, sliding it against Amber's skin, freeing it from bondage. Ouch!

This had been a part of her breast for 59 days and she had taken such good care with cleaning it, never getting an infection like so many other patients did. Meticulous and ritual-like in her daily regimen, this apparatus was now cast aside as if it were old fishing line from an ancient reel. We both stared at it in the trashcan, not sure whether to hold a sacred burial or burn the damn thing. Finally Amber sat up, feeling slightly nauseous, looking rather pale. I placed a cold, wet cloth to her forehead trying to soothe her final ordeal. That was that. With a slight apology for causing her pain, the assistant didn't even tell us her name, and then she was gone.

Friday, May 10, 1996

We are home for good! No longer prisoners of the village, we are free to enjoy the simple pleasures of our home. Along with the perks comes a much faster paced lifestyle. Bridgett is busier than usual because she is now a cheerleader (hooray!) and practices with the squad have added to her already full school schedule and dance company rehearsals. I am proud of the way she is juggling her time and still finding some to spend with her sister.

Putting the past behind us has been a struggle as the worrisome pain Amber feels in her neck is ever present. I've been trying to play it down, but it is wearing me out. A visit with her doctor is forthcoming and maybe he can put her mind at ease with a simple explanation. She is quite tearful and depressed. I suspect some of it is due to the morphine withdrawal. Maybe he can put her on an anti-depressant to combat the downward spiral she seems to be on. I swear it is always something. At least we are on our own home court and I have some back up players to help out.

Thursday, May 9, 1996

Last night the AGHS Dance Company had their annual performance and Bridgett choreographed and performed a ballet dance especially for Amber. It was beautifully done to the music of Sinead O'Connor. Her friends Tahirah and Staci danced with her and it was the most touching thing I've ever seen her do for her sissy. There wasn't a dry eye in the house, even Dr. Dan shed a tear, confessing it later after it was over. It was truly a memorable experience for our family, and as Amber and I huddled together, I had my head close to hers, our tears blended together in a harmony of happiness.

Chapter Twenty-five

Quality of life

Wednesday, May 22, 1996

 The mystery of the "phantom pain" in Amber's neck has been solved; Shingles. Aka: herpes zoster virus. This is one helluva way to recuperate after all she has been through. Her completely hairless head is now speckled with a trail of sores leading downward to the side of her neck to the place where the pain was stemming from in early diagnosis. Now it is the cause for this less serious disease, but nonetheless one to be reckoned with.

 The nerve endings are alive with fire where the buggers are erupting into open sores like the chicken pox of her childhood years. A most debilitating setback to renewed socialization; Amber is now situated on the couch, dotted with white zovirex ointment on each infected site, refusing to venture out nor allowing any visitors in. It's just as well. They would not like her company right now.

 I have given up my pep talks for the time being and settled for merely listening. This has been a huge test of my patience and love for my sweet daughter. Remembering the dozens of baths I gave her when she was eight and covered head to foot with the damn things, this really wasn't so bad. Amber would disagree, I'm sure.

 And what of Bridgett? She has fled the infirmary for distant places, usually driving around with her friends, doing everything but studying. Her senior year is anything but typical considering the health of her sibling. I understand the dilemma, but failing school now would be a disaster. And upon being told she is burning the candle at both ends I get the favorite retort, "Whatever…"

Tom has been forced to seek work out of town. This is creating an additional burden on me. Not only are we running out of money, my role as the happy homemaker is turning into heavy ball breaker. Being the only parent around all week is not winning me a popularity contest. My nerves are frazzled and I see no end in sight to our current troubles. I am planning on going on strike or considering a part time job to help make ends meet if he doesn't find work here soon. Come to think of it, a job might give me some rest and the money would help, too.

There is no point in dwelling on the black cloud hovering over our house. I refuse to let this get me down. After all, there is much to be grateful for. Amber is cancer-free. That says it all. In this grand scheme of things, that is of utmost importance. She has come a long way and even though this setback is unwanted, it is not life threatening, nor is the money thing. So, we tighten up our belts, accept charitable donations from our church that seem to come at the right times, and we pray for Amber's durable remission. I have learned to prioritize my worry machine.

Camp Reach for the Stars is the end of the month and hopefully Amber will feel well enough to attend. This will be our second one and two of the nurses that volunteer for the weekend's activities are ones from Dr. Dan's office. Ann, lovingly nicknamed "Red" by our family, and Faith Ann, are the best camp counselors around. We never worry about Amber's health because they are on site and Dr. Dan will be there again as camp doctor. Bridgett's senior prom is on the same weekend, but it is so important to connect with other families that are dealing with cancer we will work that conflict out when the time comes.

Our little Elena is steadily recuperating from her BMT and has had two favorable C.A.T. scans. She and her family will be attending camp this year. I look forward to seeing them on good circumstances. Being out in nature will be very healing for our families.

Monday, June 3, 1996

Camp was a great success. We had the nicest surprise when we arrived. The pediatric nurse at French Hospital known by all as "Ped's Pati" was assigned to our cabin and she had decorated it with tiny white lights and cute furnishings from her home. Flowers, wallpaper, and various niceties adorned our nest and Amber was delighted. It was most quaint and unlike the other rustic cabins. It also had a small heater and inside plumbing. This was a real treat meant to honor Amber for her bravery in the cancer war zone. Because she was still frail and marginally neutropenic, our family was situated right next to Dr. Dan. We felt like royalty.

I worked out the prom dilemma by fixing Bridgett's hair at camp on Saturday morning and she left on her own to attend the ball. Once again I succeeded in being in two places at once. Don't all mom's learn how to do this by the time their children are teenagers?

If children have to get cancer, this camp is a resting place along the way. An oasis in the barren land of needle sticks, chemo and C.T. scans. The family truly gets a rest from the horrible world they have been engulfed in. For three days and two nights, the respite the parents get while the nurse volunteers take care of their loved ones is priceless. We always came away richer for having had the weekend, and sad as it was to leave, worth the effort by far.

Chapter Twenty-six

Grim Reaper

Monday, June 17, 1996

    Dr. Dan just called me. Erin died this morning. My heart is hurting. I'm asking, " Why?" We just saw her walk across the stage to receive her high school diploma and spent an evening with her family watching her open her presents. Amber had to help her as she was very weak and couldn't do it for herself. I'm so grateful we were able to be there with her. It proves what we have learned through our ordeal; each day we must live for this one only so we have no regrets. But, her life was over too soon.

    As a mother I can't stop crying and there is a deep pain in my chest. Robin must be devastated. I long to call her and just tell her I love her and how sorry I am that her baby girl is gone. She fought so valiantly, tried so hard to live. Like the wind that grows into a terrible storm, destroying as it builds in intensity, then suddenly, it is gone and what's left is a memory of the intense drama and crisis and a quiet stillness and an incredible sense of loss for the way it was before the storm hit.

    I can't forget Erin's face, sunken in at her temples, her legs only bone, sitting in the wheelchair, no use of her right hand, a constant pain in her young eyes turned old and cold, begging her dad to take her home, yet thanking us for giving her a present, a little pin that made her laugh. It said, "I'm having such a marvelous time, now I think

I'll throw up." The kind of humor only cancer survivors can get the true sardonic meaning of.

Amber is taking this well, maybe it has even gotten her to think how she must choose to go on, when the conversation we had only a month ago had her doubting if she could handle another recurrence. And she had given up inside and told me if these were her last days she wanted to spend them with her family. I am now seeing a small change in her demeanor. She has been cleaning out her room and looking at her old yearbooks. She is in a transition period of acceptance of being well and allowing herself the right to look to the future.

The memorial service was long. Dr. Dan stood between my girls as the preacher spoke. It was so very hard to look at the casket and believe what was really happening. The day was sunny, crisp, and breezy in Los Osos and there was a wonderful showing of friends to support the family. I could see Robin going through the motions, holding it together with thread. I didn't want to know how that felt. This was too close for comfort...not in proximity, but in knowing that any one of us that battled this dreaded disease could be in the same situation.

For Robin

Let's dream of a place——
where pain's no more
and Erin runs free and smiles galore
Let me take you there
you deserve a rest
you've labored so hard
put to the test
your shadow gone
but not forgotten
her voice a song in the darkest night
The pain is real, yet you cannot feel
Too soon to heal
Let me take you there
And hold you tight
And let you cry into the night
And tell you its gonna' be alright
Let me take you there
Her star is bright

June 17, 1996
Janine

Chapter Twenty-seven

One has to be down to get back up

Monday, June 10, 1996

    I write in my journal tonight because I feel so alone. I stopped writing because I was tired of spewing out the technical details of my life, tired of my need to outline what I did each day and catch up what had taken place up to that point. Now, I write only to release the many feelings I am unable to voice everyday.

    It has been over two years since this journey began and while I am thankful for all of my numerous blessings, I am at a point where I'm tired of feeling so alone. This disease has slowly taken away those people whom I had to help me feel young and spontaneous. I am no longer the one Sandra calls to go out and drink or party with. I am now labeled as fragile and a "safe afternoon lunch" type of friend. "Save my night plans for Hilda who is more fun, not such a drag."

    People no longer call to see how I am and what I've been up to. They are afraid to ask for fear I may tell them all the gruesome details. I'm a safe movie date once a month for Todd, who claims to worry about me yet he hasn't spoken to me in over a month. Monica is all the way in San Francisco carrying on with her new life, meeting friends, and even dating a guy she met on the BART. My life goes on unchanging with exception to how I am physically. That's about as unpredictable as it gets.

My highlights for the day are planting flowers, playing with my cat, running some errands usually to pick up some prescriptions and once a week to get a blood draw. My nights consist of Must See TV, NBC. I figured out I that I watch about 28 hours a week which is entirely too much. It's about the only thing that I've found keeps me from feeling sorry for myself lately. I pray to God each night for some happiness. All I want is to have a friend to hang out with that is someone outside of my family.

My Mom has become my bestest friend in the whole world, but I am entirely too dependent on her. It wasn't until this week that I realized just how much. She has been in N.M. since Saturday and I've found I am lost. I spend almost every moment with her and now that she's absent I don't feel that I have direction.

All of my friends from high school have evolved into individuals with lives unique to the rest. They have met new friends, found boyfriends or girlfriends, are close to graduating from college, some have kids. Regardless of the path, they each have made decisions as to where they want to be. Me…I have had most of my choices taken away. I've adjusted and accepted each obstacle thrown at me, but only because I have to. Each month that has past has pushed me further and further from where I would like to be right now. Ideally I would like to see myself at the present with friends, a romantic opportunity, close to my bachelor's (degree) and most of all happy. Instead, I am friendless, a loner, boyfriendless, working on a few units here and there (at the community college) and extremely depressed and lonely. For my health I know that I must get out of this negative dump, I only pray that God sends me a miracle!!!

Chapter Twenty-eight

<u>A friend indeed</u>

Tuesday, June 25, 1996

This month is going by so slowly. Our finances don't warrant a vacation, but my school loan does. We are planning a "victory" trip to Albuquerque by way of Disneyland. Once Amber is feeling tip top, we will make our way to the Magical Kingdom followed by the Land of Enchantment. If we don't do it now, it will be put off until next year and we all feel we deserve a special vacation after all we have been through.

Amber had her own excitement come by way of her ex-boyfriend, Todd. He invited her to attend the Garth Brooks concert with him in Los Angeles. This was the best thing to happen to her since I don't know when. She was so thrilled! Dad took her to buy some Wranglers and she was set to go. My heart was full when I saw her smile ear to ear. She was finally doing something young and spontaneous. Thank you, Todd. You hit the mark.

She would have some good, solid memories of something besides medical tests, scans and needle pokes. Next time Sandra comes over, look out! There will be some great stories to tell of her all night date with Todd and Garth.

Monday, July 1, 1996

Ok, it's a new month, finally. Sunny weather, no fog and Amber and I have been gardening in the back yard. The physical therapy is good for both of us. She is pulling out of her depression and the shingles are a thing of the past. One more dreaded trip to City of Hope for a routine exam was made more pleasant by Angel Flights, a program of volunteer pilots who transport patients to major medical centers in California. Our three-hour trip by car was cut down to one, and the view of the coastline was breathtaking. Amber, Bridgett, and myself were passengers on our first flight ever in a single engine plane. Thanks to John Webster and Jerry Johnson, I didn't have to drive all day long.

The visit was successful in many ways. Bridgett was finally able to meet some of the people and live through a day in Amber's life at a major medical center. By mid-day, she must have been overwhelmed. During Amber's routine blood draw, she began to cry. At last her feelings were coming out and she was able to let go of the brave façade she had been hiding behind. It was a real bonding experience for these two sisters. I watched in awe as I felt the experience change them both for the better.

The trip back home was uneventful, save the method of travel. We were exhausted from the trip, not only the traveling part, the emotional, too. We had some time to talk about our upcoming trip and it was decided we will go to Disneyland, the Joffrey Ballet performance of Romeo and Juliet in L.A., visit relatives in Albuquerque, then on the way home the Grand Canyon the scene of the crime, where our honeymoon took place. Next thing in order is to have a giant yard sale to earn the money to go. Where there's a will, there's a way.

True Grit

And in this corner,
        weighing 109 lbs
        a tower of power at 5 ft 2 inches
Ladies and gentlemen
        this blonde bomber
        equipped with a
        full-time smile
        and enough experience and tenacity
        to shatter the confidence
        of any worthy opponent

The crowd cheers
She dances around the ring
        with sheer determination
        shows no fear
        knows where the ropes are
        and looks stealthily at her nemesis
Sizing it up
        saying a prayer
        disregarding the enormity
        of its strength and power
Yet she goes in
        and takes the first punch

She reels from the first blow
        clearing her head
        her coach assesses the damage
Still shaken, and weaker
        the ever -present smile
        takes form over her lips
A break in the action
        allowing her a brief respite
        from the beating she's taken

Round two
        comes too quickly

She gathers her strength
        and forges ahead
Staying low, eyes steady
        A bit more cautious
The memory of the last blow
        fresh in her mind
Somewhere deep inside
        inner strength renewed
She asks for help
        from above
She ducks and maneuvers
        her small frame
        gets nabbed, but bounces back
The sweat is flowing
        A staggering blow
        to the mouth
        the gut
Her body cries out in pain
        She's wrung out and so tired
                so tired

A voice from the coach
        "keep dancin"
        she makes round two
        her body exhausted
        her spirit alive
With all that is left
she lands a blow
        and with breath heaving
        skin torn and burning
she scores the knockout punch
and stands alone
victorious

                Janine

Chapter Twenty-nine

On the road again

Friday, July 12, 1996

Our kickoff for our ten-day family vacation was a success. Disneyland will never be the same, nor will we. We took in every possible ride, watched the Electric Light Parade (it's farewell performance) and closed the place down. I never worried about Amber or how tired she was or wasn't and I don't think she did either. It was so exciting to be somewhere besides a hospital.

There appears to be an adjustment period needed for Tom and Bridgett, as they are getting on each other's nerves, but other than that we are enjoying being together as a family again. We have all been under our own kind of strain the past few months, but agree a road trip was the best way to let that go.

The ballet performance was captivating and even Tom had to admit it was well done. One of the selections was done to the music of Prince and got the girls' attention for sure. Our motel stay was quite restful. An entire day was spent laying by the pool, soaking up the sun, swimming, reading and napping. Now it was an official vacation.

No matter how you try to break up the miles, traveling to and half way through N.M. is boring and seems like an eternity. Finally seeing the Sandia Mountains was a relief. As they lay in front of us like the dark blue hem of a wide skirt, I felt as I always do; we were home.

My niece, Christine, gave us a barbecue at her beautiful home, and Amber was the guest of honor. Although that was the last thing she wanted to be, she graciously mingled, let people touch her fuzzy baldhead and put up with hoards of wanted and unwanted attention. I neglected to realize just how tired she had become, and when we retired to our motel the tears were abundant. She abhorred the pitiful glances she saw on people's faces and just wished for one thing, to be normal again. The transition from being quite hermit-like and sequestered in the hospital environment, then more of the same in our own quiet home had given her a false sense of security. Now in the wide-open world, she wished to regress back into the comfortable folds of her own small family. I had to admit I was out of my comfort zone as well. We decided being around the multitude of well-wishers was over; that the remainder of our stay would be spent in intimate settings with a limited number of extended family present. First stop, Aunt Joan's, a safe haven.

Tuesday, June 16, 1996

It is time for our departure, and as sad as I am to say goodbye to my family, I am relieved to go. The harshness of people's reaction to Amber is beginning to dim, or maybe the novelty has worn off. Admittedly, she has been the topic of conversation here for the last two years. I made sure Amber's Angels got frequent updates on her condition, current methods of treatment, good news, and bad news. When they got to see her they wanted to touch her, and know she was finally all right. I don't blame anyone for scrutinizing her. She is a beautiful miracle and they were all asked to partake in the prayers that made her so. In the years to come Amber will learn to appreciate the way she brought everyone together through prayer and love.

In the days to come, when I reminisce about the Grand Canyon portion of our trip, I will fondly think of Bridgett sitting in the back seat of the hot car, stubbornly refusing to get out to see the Petrified Forest. "Just a bunch of dirt and weeds and old wood. Where's the telephone? I want to go home and be with my friends." Ah, teenagers.

BOOK FOUR

LAST DAYS

Last days
In my home
All I want to do
Is be at peace
Tell dad
I'll be OK
Don't worry, mom
Love, Amber
~This is a good day to die~

Chapter One

Relapse

Tuesday, August 13, 1996

    The night was long. I had spoken to Dr. Dan late. Everyone in the house was asleep but me. The information he divulged to me was for my ears only. It would change our lives forever.

    My mind went to instant prayer. I began bargaining with God. "If you would just change your mind, no one will ever know." I had offered silence of the words I had heard, if he would just take them back. I honestly believed it would work. I had such a belief in the power of prayer, I stayed up for hours after that phone call and made sure I backed up my deal with a concrete, down on my knees, crying to the pit of my soul, covenant.

    I was begging for my daughter's life. Begging for mercy. In the darkness of the night I had humbled myself and offered anything to have that cup taken away from her.

Interlude

"I can't move." The all-consuming fear bubbled up from my toes. I remember feeling frozen, my feet in cement. There I was, perched on the side of a steep mountain covered in loose dirt and gravel, nary a tree in sight. Below there was only the deep, threatening to drown me if I fell, blue water, above more slippery gravel, steep and threatening as far as my eye dared see.

As if wearing blinders, I refused to move my head at first, then upon partial recovery from my fear, recollected my sweet babies. One on either side of me, climbing in a chain while daddy forged ahead alone. I heard them crying, "Mommy, what's wrong?" but I couldn't budge. Then a new terror reached my brain. The old phobia lingered beneath my consciousness; all three of us falling into the water below and me unable to save my drowning children.

An eternity passed as I went in and out of near, but quiet hysteria. I was the charge for this eight and five-year old. They were clinging to me for dear life and I was helpless to save them.

My body was numb with the exception of feeling my girl's hands in mine. That connection would eventually bring me back to a long enough period of sanity to let go of them one at a time so their father could walk them to safety. Once they were on safe ground upon the cliff above, he came back to retrieve what was left of me. As I awaited my knight in shining armor, I began to pray with every fiber of my being, "Please watch over my daughters until we are safely together again."

As if in a daze, step by step, I let myself be led by my husband up the to the lesser of two evils, the precipice overlooking the dreadful lake. I felt like a lamb being led by its mother, every step gingerly made in trepidation, and the lingering fear, now foremost, of my children above falling down into the abyss of water below. The utter terror of being helpless to save them permeating my thoughts, and a gnawing pain of knowing I failed them.

Chapter Two

<u>God throws another curve ball</u>

Tuesday, August 13, 1996

  Life for me is an intense roller coaster and lately it is filled with many low dips. I now have found out that my chemo isn't working and the disease has popped up in (near) my lung. I feel that I'm running out of options and I'm terrified at what that means. I know that death is part of life, but I don't think I've lived a full life. I have so much left to experience, I swear I have a black cloud following me wherever I go. Just when I think that things are getting bearable, God throws me another curve ball. I'm so tired of fighting to keep faith that I'm going to beat this thing. Not only do I feel that this disease is ruling me, I feel that my life is no longer mine.

  I'm unsure of where I belong. My world consists of medical issues and my family. My parents have to worry about who will be home with me if they want to go out on a date and I feel guilty for not allowing them to have their own life. I've continued to tell myself that this is happening for a "reason," but what more could I possibly gain from this continued situation?

  I keep feeling more and more closed in and trapped. I have no escape to take me away from the constant reminder that I am ill. I am <u>so</u> frustrated with my lack of control over this situation. I need God to tell me where to go from here and how do I beat this monster that is sucking the life out of me? If I have to live with this sucker for the rest of my life then help me *to live without holding back.*

I feel so overwhelmed with my circumstances and I'm having trouble verbalizing what I'm feeling. I have a very important decision that needs to be made and it will affect my life. What will be the next choice for treatment and will it be the "right" choice?

Fear

"I'm scared," she said
uncertain why
"I'm scared," she said
"I'm going to die"
they poke and prod
cut here to here
there's nothing left
just plain, pure fear
I cannot cry
I'm swirling, lost
not giving up
but at what cost?
My life a series
of operations
unknown treatments
radiations
Insane I feel
from all this waiting
terror filled
anticipating
Hurry up
my faith
is fading

Janine

Chapter Three

<u>De'ja-vu</u>

Wednesday, August 28, 1996

     I have been here before. It is City of Hope village and not much has changed. Maybe a little less hope on my part. I just took a crying shower after our visit with Dr. Spyberg. He was so serious, but what else is new? The parts I hated were the "likelihood that Amber's cancer will return after the forthcoming planned radiation." The litany of his lecture included the obvious facts that her relapses have come shortly after treatment each time, making a cure sound unlikely. "But, I have a patient with active Hodgkin's who goes to work each day." I'm sorry, but I want a little more for my daughters' future. He also mentioned having Bridgett HLA typed for a possible donor related (allogeneic) bone marrow transplant down the line. Oh, God.

     What about immunotherapy, I wondered? I had done my homework and read about the use of one's own immune system to tame the beast. Bingo! Here was something discussed by him and his colleagues as a method of treatment following the scheduled radiation of her right chest cavity. This new site is close to her lung. Again our favorite surgeon, Dr. Howard, performed the most recent of her many intrusive procedures; a biopsy of a node affected under her armpit verified the cancer was back.

     I'm tired of them mapping out the pattern so defined as one of the classic differences of Hodgkin's disease versus Non-Hodgkin's disease. The supposition that makes the type she has more curable than the other. But there are those who slip through the cracks, who fall in the 25% that relapse from the "good type" of cancer to have. Good defined as easier to combat and cure. I find the word blasphemous. Here is a young woman, barely 20 years of age with the "good" type of cancer. Bullshit.

So we have taken to the world wide web in search of new options that don't involve cutting it out, burning it out, or poisoning it out, aka surgery, radiation, chemotherapy. With the information comes statistics that are at best disheartening. With only a 25% chance a second BMT will work, now her numbers are reversed. What is the good in that?

All these facts and what am I feeling? Like my God has deserted us in our hour of need. Like my child's world is being attacked by a pack of rabid dogs and I have no weapon to save her except my love and voice. So be it. If I can't kill the bastards, I'll just detour them for the time being. My own way is staying involved with the health care team of doctors and nurses and reminding them of the importance of their commitment to my daughter's excellent care. I have asked those serving her to pray with me for her wellness and that the present attempt will finally kill the cancer roaming around in her precious body. I asked each of them to autograph her hospital gown and make that vow to be positive and caring while treating her.

We have been going to the Wellness Community in Pasadena and receiving much help through this recent ordeal. All services, including group therapy sessions with licensed professionals are absolutely free for patients and caregivers. Meeting other people with similar situations has been so rewarding and the Tai Chi classes and speakers on meditation and relaxation has given Amber some wonderful ideas to calm her mind.

Wednesday, September 4, 1996

The bad news of my stepfather, Larry, passing away yesterday, has renewed my vigilance of getting Amber well. My dear mother, now alone, is still being positive and optimistic even in the aftermath of the death of her husband. I know where my undying hope comes from.

Waiting…

We play the waiting game
                    so well
Like standing watch 'tween earth
                    and hell
While docs play God
                    we carry on
Not faceless as they'd
                    have us be
I'm making sure her face
                    they'll see
She's bright and smiling
                    on this earth
asking for another birth

So wait we shall
                    in patience be
We'll wait and do
                    necessity
No wasted time
                    together we
share precious moments

just her
        and me

Janine
September '96

Chapter Four

Life on the outside

Sunday, September 15, 1996

      Even though Amber and I are commuting weekly down south to the hospital 200 miles away for daily radiation, and Tom is doing the same thing up north seeking employment near San Francisco, the hometown pride of the Eagles football team is keeping everyone distracted. This is mainly due to the fact that our Bridgett is now a varsity cheerleader and her main squeeze, Matt, is number 23, defensive linebacker. It makes for a wonderfully "normal" family weekend, even though we know our situation is anything but normal. We pack up blankets, hot chocolate, candy bars and lots of spirit to every weekend game, and whether they win or lose, we are happy to be a part of the whole thing.

      We have been given lemons and are doing our best to make lemonade. Bridgett is holding the fort down during the week with Monica, Amber's high school buddy, as a companion.

      The absence of both parents is taking its toll on Bridgett's grades. She is slipping and I have spoken to my dear friend and one of her teachers, Debby, to make herself available to Bridgett if she is having difficulty on any given day at school. She has permission to go visit her if things get too rough and she needs someone to talk to.

Another dear teacher from our parish, Mr. Fogarty, is helping her to complete the community service requirement needed for graduation. If it weren't for these dedicated teachers, she would be failing school and kicked off the squad and dance company. This is beginning to look like a long struggle to keep her in school, but there is hope with the help of our concerned community.

And what would we do without our friends? Karen and Wes, Julie and Greg, Dr. Dan and Mary Ellen, who are keeping an eye on her while we are struggling in separate sides of the state.

I miss my home, my husband, and my other child. I miss our life before cancer hit the fan; I miss the little things like cleaning my house, watering the flowers. I miss the good health of my first-born child. She was always active, dancing, hiking, dating, laughing, and teasing. What happened to that carefree young adult that danced on point, bravely hiked Half-Dome, and taught me to do the boot scootin' boogie? I'm terrified how this all will turn out and I don't know who to tell.

While we are being swirled around in this salad spinner called life, we try to maintain some semblance of normality. The weekends have saved us from sure doom and gloom. When we are all together, the sun seems to shine brighter, the beds are softer, and the days go by way too fast.

Monday, September 23, 1996

Amber's tumor has already gone down in size after only five radiation treatments! That is fantastic news and she deserves it. She has been feeling tired and had loss of appetite, but this gives us hope and it is all worth it. On the down side, she has been feeling some tingling down her spine and in her fingers. There is also a hacking cough that has begun to plague her night and day.

Before the radiation began, Dr. Robodeck met with us and warned Amber of possible side effects. A subcutaneous atrophy of the fat on the strip of her breast where the radiation field is will change the texture of the breast tissue and make it appear different than the other one. Also the chance of a modest amount of lung damage, and rib fracture is possible. Unfortunately, there was some overlapping necessary to get the entire tumor. He gave her the option to avoid the lung, but she decided to go ahead and do whatever was needed to save her life. Not an easy decision to make for a 20 year old, but it had to come from her.

I am fearful of the chipping away of her dignity. Throughout these procedures, I have been vigilant about keeping her covered as much as possible, making sure the techs make her as comfortable as can be, and playing some soothing music as I massage her feet in readiness of the actual radiation treatment. I then stand outside the door of the radiation room, praying the rays target is successfully eradicating the enemy. She has started calling her good cells "Pac-Man," and visualizes them to eating up the cancer cells one at a time until they are all gone.

Chapter Five

Dr. Doom

Tuesday, October 1, 1996

Our visit with Dr. Spyberg was less than stellar. I made the mistake of asking him how Amber's case compared to others he has had that were similar. He had to say that there is a good chance the cancer that is shrinking will come back once radiation is completed. He couldn't comment on how much time that would take, but he was very stoic and matter-of-fact in his vagueness. While we were trying to swallow this he also said he doubted she could have any more chemo because it would do more harm than good. Did I hear him correctly? I was shaking. We had just been given supposed good news the tumor was shrinking, and now he was giving her a death sentence. I was in shock and Amber was numb.

As we walked back to the village, she bravely said she doesn't agree with him, but it bothers her that he talks that way. Sometimes I get so scared. I want to cry, hide, then I see her smile and she looks so normal I just can't believe it can be that grim.

We decided to take in a meeting at the Wellness center and bring up what her doctor said in our individual groups. Almost everyone suggested we change doctors. No shit.

With only one more visit scheduled with him, Amber decided not to rock the boat. After this, she would be released back to Dr. Dan anyway, so she just preferred to let it go. I didn't want to let it go. I wanted to punch him in the nose. I did the next best thing. I sent him an anonymous poison poem.

Dr. Doom

There once was a doctor of doom
That's how he came out of the womb
His logic and facts
Made you feel like the axe
Was about to descend on the room

One day with his usual gloom
While his patient did sit in the room
No smile on his face
No hope—not a trace
Proceeded his litany of doom

"Your cup is half empty, not full
if you think you are well, think again
start accepting your fate
sit right down here and wait
your positive thinking's insane!"

Well, the patient slipped off of the table
Her HOPE kept her healthy and able
She knew she felt well
She had broken his spell
And that is the end of the fable

Chapter Six

<u>Trouble brewing</u>

December 1996

    My entire family has "dis-ease." It is a rampant illness that is so contagious you can get it over the telephone. It is so widely spread even my relatives in Albuquerque have it, a thousand miles away. Every person I remotely know has it from the cable man to the postal clerk, the bank teller to the grocery produce man. It permeates my being, wakes me up in the middle of the night, and takes my breath away. What causes it? Cancer. How do you get it? From worrying your brains out. How do you get rid of it? You don't. Can you live with it? Yes, if you call that living. Is it expensive? Damn right. Is there hope? I certainly hope so.

    Between Tom's unemployment and my inability to get a job, we are sinking into a large pit of quicksand. He has taken off work so much to be home for tests, treatments, results of C.A.T. scans, etc., and gets no pay for no work, our pockets are near empty. Now, I know people say money isn't everything, and I would agree if I had some. Standing in line in the rain at the Harvest Bag to get a sack of donated groceries for two-fifty, isn't my idea of fun. Never mind the humiliation. I lost that a long time ago. A mother takes care of her children.

"In a desperate attempt to set the world's Guinness Book of Records, the Carter family had yet another yard sale—shooting for the record of 500, Mrs. Carter, wearily smiling, holding her back, wearing her masking tape bracelet, and firmly clutching her money bag, was heard giving professional advice to her daughter, Amber."

"Don't let them take anything unless you set the price. You have control, don't be pushed around, be assertive—$2.00 wasn't too much for the radio, if they argue, double the price!"

Her legacy is left to her children. When she died, her epitaph read, "When the going got rough, she had a yard sale."

I learned a long time ago without humor we are all sunk. It came to pass that when my sense of it went so far downhill, I considered suicide. I figured it was a small sacrifice, but the $25,000 life insurance policy I had would pull them out of a jam and they'd be better off without me and with the money. I mean when that yard sale yielded a whopping $43, and we started using Amber's credit card to pay our bills, and I knew we were in real trouble.

Tom took the $43 to go out of town again to find work, leaving me alone again and setting off more deep depression. It is with great relief that even though I got to the point of planning my demise to look like an accident, I finally sought help from a therapist and got on anti-depressants. Looking back, I now realize how sick I had become. I even thought he could start a new life with a younger woman, and my insurance money would help him start his own business. I would have some peace in the knowledge I could do something by dying. After all, we must die sometime, right? Why not do it and leave your family better off? Nuts! I was certifiable.

When the anti-depressants began to kick in, I had renewed strength to go on and get back in the fight. I started looking into alternative methods of fighting cancer. Acupuncture for her cough and any pain or nausea, herbal remedies such as Floressence, Esiac, Ginseng, and marijuana tea for anti-oxidants and loss of appetite due to chemo/radiation. Reiki therapy for mind control in healing was a great relaxing tool for Amber. She even took classes and received her own certificate for performing Reiki on herself. I made sure she meditated every day and used positive imagery tapes to relax and rejuvenate her spiritual side. We exercised regularly together doing a routine we had made up incorporating dance, weight watchers, aerobics, and even western line dancing. We would giggle and sometimes lapse into the swing, me playing the boy and twirling her around on my finger the way Todd used to. My friend, Ann, gave us private yoga lessons in her living room for free and we learned more meditation techniques doing the "corpse" pose. This was good for stretching the body and mind. We all needed that.

What we didn't need was the news we got after the scheduled C.A.T. scan. It wasn't time for Amber to be cancer free yet.

Chapter Seven

<u>The dragon rears its ugly head</u>

Thursday, December 12, 1996

The same original site behind the sternum was again the culprit. For all my and thousands of peoples' prayers and faith in God's divine plan, I do NOT understand why she has to endure more pain and suffering and that her life's plans had to be put on hold <u>one more time.</u>

No early present for Christmas. The disease remains alive and growing within her chest. I wish I could reach in and yank it out or pound on it with my fist until it screams out for mercy. How merciful has it been to Amber? Those damn cells cruising around in her body need to be burned out once and for all. Unfortunately along with their demise goes good cells and healthy tissue. Some choice she has. The choices are becoming fewer and fewer and now that is a new and terrifying worry. I won't go to that place. I must stay in today and focus on the plan being formulated by the doctors we trust. I guess Dr. Doom was right. Damn him! It's been two years and I feel we are right back where we started.

Tom took the news very hard and cried a lot. At least he's not mad at God or Dr. Dan this time. He's just sad for Amber. It's hard for him because he just can't "fix" it and make it better. Pain is inevitable, suffering is optional and by the end of the day we were all in acceptance, including Amber. She is so very wise, and so very hopeful. Bridgett was her "sissy" and joked around with her and held her hand and it helped so much to have her with us. We are one unit against the evil that has picked on us for too long. I'm not giving up. Nor is Amber.

She went to visit her therapist the following day, and by using her session, was bombarded with information about a doctor in Mexico she thought she should see. This was totally out of her realm of therapy. She had clearly overstepped her professional boundaries. Amber came home crying and I had to call and put her in her place, also firing her. That was the kookiest suggestion we had received for a cure since someone had mentioned going to a clinic in Arizona to receive "elephant's milk."

As bad as those options sound, when Dr. Dan called me at my temporary job at the bank and told me the next step for her would be more systemic poisoning, I was numb. When the full effect of the repercussions of more chemo settled into my brain, the flood of tears and pain turned my face inside out. The world had cracked and the oceans just washed over me. It was up to me to tell Amber the news.

When I got home I just couldn't face her. The next day Todd was taking her to Magic Mountain and she was so excited to be going somewhere with a young friend. I let it pass. It could keep the secret inside the safe of my hardened heart until tomorrow. Go and play, my darling, and be young for a day.

The next morning Amber came in to greet her dad and I in our bed. Her usual smile and lovely morning disposition was cuddled alongside us and we were a cozy threesome, just like when she was a baby and would crawl into bed with us. Joy in the morning! I wanted to make this moment stretch as long as I could, but aloud she wondered why the doctor hadn't called her yet about their decision for treatment protocol. I hated this so much, then Tom took over and told her the truth about the chemo. It was the first time he had been the bad news breaker. Before we knew it, Bridgett had joined us and we were all crying together. I had to get up and stiffen that upper lip of mine. I had my grief yesterday and now was ready for the next phase of the new plan to rid her of the evil lurking in her chest.

Later on in the day, Dr. Dan called Amber and after their lengthy conversation I went in to her bedroom where she was lying down, crying. He had given her the statistics of her survival. Something like one in ten chance for a response. Was he crazy? What the f_ _ _! She was devastated and just laid there as if to say, "What's the use?" He may as well have put a gun to her head and played Russian roulette. I calmed her down by giving her an analogy of her as a dancer and her partner drops her. What would be her options? 1. Tell the partner to get lost. 2. Tell him how she feels and not to drop her again. 3. Quit the dance. She smiled and said she wanted to continue dancing and she would talk to her partner about <u>never </u>dropping her again!

On Christmas Eve I got an early present. I saw Amber get up on her hind legs and fight for her rights and her dignity. She is truly becoming a victor and not a victim. Dr. Dan called and she actually had the courage to tell him how she felt about his statistics. When she was done she seemed to stand taller and by telling him she didn't want to hear any more of his numbers unless she asks for them, she became empowered before my very eyes. She also <u>told</u> him her intentions of incorporating alternative therapies along with his conventional ones. She stood victorious! He will treat her with more respect now, and even told her to "stay feisty." Hooray for you, Amber. You have opened a new chapter in your life. I am so proud of you.

As the year draws to a close, we haven't much that is positive to say about 1996. Christmas will come and go and we will try to get through to the next obstacle of trying to save our daughter from the clutches of the beast.

Chapter Eight

A new year

Sunday, January 5, 1997

It's a new year with more challenges and renewed hope. Amber's newfound assertiveness and determination to be well, against the odds, is infectious. We need to bolster our bravery, battle down the hatches, and follow her lead.

Shattering my sense of fairness is the alarming news of our Elena's relapse. At the age of six she should be playing happily at school, but instead her parents are considering a move to New York to participate in a clinical trial to save her life. The type of cancer she has is rare. How much punishment can her little body take?

In our own household, Amber has had a new port-a-cath inserted just beneath the surface of the skin on her breast by Dr. Howard. Just two days ago it was placed and already tomorrow she receives her first session of the new chemo drug selected by her team of doctors to be administered at Dr. Dan's office. Last night before going to bed, I gave her communion and she smiled and said, "This is a new beginning." How brightly she looked at me as if she were getting ready for a trip, or a special date. How can I be doubtful or sad with her smiling, hopeful face? I am amazed at her ability to turn this into thoughts of a new beginning…she really is my strength and I shall do whatever I can to help her get through this.

Along with this new chemo will come more hair loss. She has accepted this unpreventable fact, but also decided to get another shorter pixie style wig to match her current hairdo. Our favorite hairstylist, Becka, has been doing some cute things with Amber's hair since the BMT, and now with the destined alopecia, comes plan B. Bridgett has already volunteered to buzz her sissy's head this time. It is always better to have a plan when it comes to this part. At least she can regain some control over part of her life.

As far as finances go, we are close to having our house repossessed. Two payments behind and the wolf is at the door. I have been working steady for the temp agency, but my wage is not enough to make a sizeable difference. Tom's work has been so sporadic, plus having to take off without pay so much is finally catching up with us. We sold our Bronco, and have received help from family members at Christmas time. Mom is always one we can count on for cash in time of need. She doesn't want me to worry about money with Amber's health being so bad. We've borrowed on the girl's life insurance policies and mine, but there is so much catching up to do. I am praying now for an end to this crisis. The most important thing right now is to get Amber well.

Meanwhile, she is enrolled in college and energized to begin. She knows she can whittle away her general education here and transfer those credits to a university at a later date. Her cough has become chronic and it makes it hard for her to walk very far, so she finally gave in and got a handicap card for her car. It was a struggle, but she only uses it for school parking which is intolerable at best. Now she loves her "handy" and can count on a parking space at all times.

Having school to look forward to has put her in a good place mentally. One of her classes is Statistics and she loves it. She doesn't take after me, that's for sure! The main thing is having purpose and responsibility. When her friends, Todd and Jess, came over to visit she had something besides cancer to talk about.

It is hard to admit, but I think she is learning to live with the disease. I still pray for the cure, and never lose hope, but the truth is she has had this for two years now and not much more than a few months without it. I have to rethink my dreams for her daily. Just to have her cancer free is at the top of the list. To find true love is next, and career goals last. She is interested in becoming a therapist so she can use her experience to help young adults going through what she has.

They say what doesn't kill you makes you stronger. Amber is a shining example of this quote.

Chapter Nine

<u>Living with cancer</u>

Tuesday, February 18, 1997

This year is well on its way. A local job for Tom has made our lives more manageable. No longer do I have to pretend I'm not home when someone comes to the door. We had a visitor from the bank checking up to see if we still lived there and hadn't skipped out. That was scary.

Amber's chemo is going slowly this time due to low hemoglobin counts making the time between treatments longer. At first she was concerned, but Dr. Dan assured her that the length between therapies was no big deal. She just will have it eight times a year instead of twelve. She was ok with that and has moved on. In fact, she said she is quite content and happy with her life right now. I am in awe. There is a certain sense of security while on chemo. It is not the waiting game played for anticipated remission or a "cure" after treatments. It is the best that can be done right now and she has chosen to go along with it. I am fiercely proud of her. She is my role model.

It is oddly comforting that we don't have to go through the larger more traumatic ordeals right now. With her in treatment, it is almost our version of normal. Our family is going on with life. Looking back at the frenzied times of surgeries, biopsies, stem cell collections, times we were torn apart by distance. When transfusion is necessary it is one of the least invasive and really just a detour of one's day. Like having a hiccough compared to a heart attack. I still have arguments with my teenager about the same things other families do. We still have activities, jobs, (thank you, God) and plans for what we'll do this summer. They are just slightly different, having to coincide with chemotherapy sessions, transfusions, and hair loss. No big deals.

Sunday, March 2, 1997

It's been a long hard week filled with crisis. Amber had chemo on Tuesday and it knocked her on her ass. She spent much time throwing up and finally got a prescription from the doc for the anti-emetic, Zofran, which helped a lot. On Wednesday, she went to class, came home and her temp was 102. Since her local doc was non-committal as to the cause, I called City of Hope and spoke to a doc there. He said it sounded like the chemo was attacking the H.D. cells causing the fever. I also called Spyberg and he said the ARA-C (chemo) sometimes can bring on fever. Who do I believe? Does it matter? She feels like shit, can't sleep, constipated, constant headache, aching of her bones, complete malaise. All I could do was give her Tylenol and validate her pain and discomfort. I hate what this stuff is doing to her. It's like seeing an alien slip into her body and take over. She gets so beat up by it, I can't bear the abuse she has to endure.

Wednesday, March 12, 1997

The worst is finally over and Amber is feeling so much better. She has been happy all week and even though her counts are low, she is full of energy once more. What an up and down month this has been. I am certain this was the chemo that made her so sick. Every two weeks or so she has to go through hell week, followed by a blood transfusion, then all over again the following month. What a way of life, but we try to make the best of it. This time her dad and I rented a movie and laid in the bed next to her. As she received the life giving blood we watched the movie together. That is truly a new kind of family bonding, a special kind of closeness.

Julie and I have been in communication a great deal lately. Elena's C.A.T. scan was neutral. No increase in tumor size but also no decrease. The eight days of constant chemo she received at Stanford only kept it from growing. My heart goes out to this brave family. Megan, her older sister, and Jamie, an older brother, are going through a rough time accepting their little sister's illness. This is so hard on the siblings. Their lives are turned upside down as well.

Chapter Ten

<u>An average, abnormal, uncommon life</u>

April-December, 1997

In my wildest dreams I would not have predicted how my life has turned out to this point. Sitting here, writing in my journal for the umpteenth time, I am at a loss for words. We have weathered many storms, and although I would have orchestrated it quite differently, it is what it is.

Two months ago I thought we were looking to begin the New Year with wellness. My intuition whispered, "cure" into my ear, but another plan was in store for Amber. It must have been "pure" for her heart remains so. Even with the odds against her, she continues to surprise everyone with the tenacity of a bulldog. If she goes under, it is only for a day at most. She feels her feelings, climbs back into the boat and sets another sail. For every setback, she has managed to turn it around. Every minus has become a plus, and each day a new beginning.

I draw my strength from this timid 20-year-old daughter of mine who has shed that persona to grow a harder, impermeable attitude of high self-esteem with the ability to change fear to hope in 24 hours. Seeing her in action, demanding she be allowed to call the shots, fills me with awe.

So many times I wanted to give up on her teenage sister, our financial dilemma, even my own life, but I trudged onward out of respect for her ability to be strong.

When friends dumped her, she was sad, but eventually was able to forgive, able to let Sandra know how she felt when she wasn't there for her, able to allow Todd to make it up to her. When the nausea became too much to bear, she bought a marijuana cook book and baked herself some special brownies to feel better. When the chemo vampire took her blood, and it took seven hours to receive a transfusion, she showed me how she could beat me at Backgammon, Monopoly and double solitaire.

College was her dream and each month she went to school she surpassed the previous one's efforts. She was on the Dean's honor roll, and continued to remain anonymous about the cancer she had. Her classmates never knew how difficult it was for her to walk from the parking lot and climb the stairs to attend classes. Attendance was paramount to her as if she were trying to prove that she was stronger and smarter than the disease that plagued her. She refused to let it rule her life as it had in the past. Here, on the campus, she could be "normal" and it was an important boost to her self-esteem, her personality and her place in the world.

Above all, she never, ever wanted pity. Don't do the pity thing, it's NO BIG DEAL!! It is what has to be done. If it is required to juggle classes with transfusions in order to stay on task, so be it. The escape of school and a place free of disease was needed, but when I would see her pale skin and fragile body getting into her car for class I just thought it was so cruel and unfair for her to suffer so much. All she wanted was to be normal.

God give me grace to help her; Mary give me compassion and patience; Holy Spirit guide me.

The day she and her dad came home with her new car, a 1995 Saturn, emerald green, her favorite color, she was radiant. Because she received a small compensation from SSI, she was able to qualify for a car loan. This was the single most adult thing she had ever accomplished on her own aside from attending college. This car meant more than transportation to her. It was a sign of a long awaited form of independence.

When Camp Reach for the Stars came in June, she was able to help with the little kids like she always wanted to do. Sort of being a camp counselor. The KSBY news channel interviewed her and she was so eloquent praising her loving family for supporting her with love and acceptance. She never made anyone feel she was doing it alone. Genuine kudos came from her lips often.

The pride she felt for her little sister was evident when she watched her receive her high school diploma. Our Baby Bridgett got through her senior year and graduated. Finally, here was some good news for the Carter clan to write home about.

Each celebration, vacation, holiday or birthday was marked with what type of therapy Amber was on and how well she felt or didn't feel. Even her dentist appointments depended on what her platelet count was. No menstrual periods allowed for the same reason, possible hemorrhaging. She had already been considered menopausal due to the high dose chemo received during the BMT.

Our lives were dictated by cancer's whims, but we worked around all of this to create our own semblance of an average, abnormal, uncommon life.

Chapter Eleven

Days of woe

January-July, 1998

    Bringing in another new year without the expectation of a cure, the realization really hit. Not only the dream of it gone out of my head, my prayers have now drastically changed to begging for my daughter's life without being cancer-free. Amber continued to do battle with new therapies, but due to the debilitating side effects thereof, such as neuropathy, migraines, heart palpitations, and continued depletion of her blood products, the more potent "cure seeking" drugs were systematically omitted. Eventually, palliative care became the method of treatment.

    Amazingly, Amber continued to walk on the treadmill, and go to her stretch class at college, determined to fight the effects and recover. Although it was a struggle, she remained very active as a group leader in the church youth group and Renew program. She also was asked to speak on behalf of Daffodil Days, an ACS fundraising event, and was interviewed at Camp again this year by KSBY. Her smile and ease at speaking in front of the camera belied her inner stage fright and she always spoke of the importance of her family in her life.

    I began working regular part time hours as a teller and wore a pager, my life - line to Amber, which cleared up my guilt for being away. However, the time away was good for both of us. She, left to her own devices, became more independent, and for a few hours a day, I could step away from the deep fears that had begun haunting me day and night about death.

Meanwhile, her sister tried out college and hated it. She opted to attend beauty school instead and had the task of going in every day for eight hours. At least I knew where she was supposed to be. Our relationship continued to unravel as her parents, or rather "the enemy." She was bent on pushing all the wrong buttons, to get attention, I suppose. It worked, even if it was the negative kind. Our desire to please her with a new car backfired. We were trying so hard, but there was much inner turmoil going on inside that teenage head. Much more than we could figure out on our own.

Our dear friends, the Macedo family temporarily relocated to New York so Elena could participate in a clinical trial there and possibly and make possibly the last valiant effort to save her life. Two months later they returned without change in the disease for the better. I feared the worst would come to pass before too long to our sweet Elena.

Sunday, August 3, 1998

It's scary to think about my sister dying. Sometimes I do think about it. She has cancer in her back now. I still don't understand why God is doing this to her. Everybody says everything happens for a reason. That was my way of justifying this disease in the beginning, but what's the reason for making her suffer for almost four years now? I can't understand. I love her so much. All I pray for is that we all have the strength to overcome any obstacle God throws at us especially her strength. (is needed)

Matt and I are doing pretty good. I am very lucky to have him in my life. I pray that we also stay strong. I love him very much.
BC

Sunday, August 9th

Yesterday was my sister's birthday. She wasn't feeling too hot. She had chemo on Thursday so she was still recuperating. I get so scared to see her weak and energy-less. I still pray for her strength. I hope and pray that God realizes how much she is needed here. I love her…
BC

Chapter Twelve

<u>Amber's Gratitude Journal</u>

August 12, 1998
     I was given this journal as a present from my cousin, Amanda, with the understanding that I would write five things I was grateful for every day. I promised that I would, but have taken a few days to motivate myself to start. (Typical procrastinator!)
     Today was a good day so I felt it was appropriate to start my journal on a positive note. Today was a beautiful sunny day. I am grateful for God blessing me with sunshine and nice weather.
Today I was blessed with an appetite. Despite radiation and the past couple of days when food was unappealing, today I had no problem eating three square meals. For this I am grateful.
I went shopping with my Mom today after radiation and spent some of my birthday $. I am thankful for the quality time I was able to spend along with my Mom.
I had a pretty full day today in which I watched very little T.V. I am grateful for the energy that allowed me to get out and about.
I am grateful for Lynn at Mission-Medical who drew my blood. It was nice not to have to worry about a second poke.

Tuesday, August 13, 1998

Today was a little frustrating to me. I was tired and felt grumpy. I can't quite put my finger on what is wrong, so it must be a combination of things. I need to find what I'm grateful for more now than ever so I can escape from this negative place. Tonight might prove to be difficult in pinpointing my five things.

I am thankful for my cozy bed that I am sitting in right now. It will bring me the sleep and rejuvenation my mind and body need.

I am grateful to have my loving cats who are so forgiving. They love me no matter what.

I am thankful for my Mom who always is there to listen to me…and give me comforting words of wisdom.

I am grateful for my Dad's job, which allows him to be home every night. I've really missed having him here.

I am thankful for my brief visit to the beach today. The ocean shows me how powerful God is and how with him anything is possible.

Wednesday, August 14, 1998

Tonight we celebrated Bridgett's birthday at the Melodrama. Today was her special day because we are leaving to visit Gram (in N.M.) on her real birthday. It was so nice to spend the evening out as a family. I have a lot to be grateful for.

I am so blessed to have a wonderful little sis whom is also my best friend. I am so thankful that we have remained close all these years.

I am thankful for parents who have been married almost 26 years. Not many people have parents who are still married. I am blessed to have two parents who love each other. I hope one day I am lucky enough to find the same long lasting relationship.

I am grateful for uplifting entertainment that allows one to forget all their troubles for a short time.

I am thankful for another day of life that was spent with those whom I love the most.

I am thankful that today is Friday. No radiation tomorrow and a whole weekend to look forward to.

Thursday, August 15, 1998

Today we went to a wedding and it wasn't until I was there that I realized how far away I am from those who I graduated with. People my age are getting married, finding careers and really moving forward to the next stage of life. I felt so distant from their world. My life has changed, but not in the way it should have. It was frustrating to talk to old acquaintances.

On the scale of their lives, I have made no accomplishments, yet in my world I have come so far and overcome so much. I couldn't even begin to explain what I've been up to the past four years, nor would they really want to know. Being surrounded by reminders of how things were and how they should be really started to get to me so I left. I guess that I have turned into a hermit. I just can't handle social situations anymore, I am happy in my cozy surroundings at home with people who care about me. Tonight in order to boost my self-esteem I decided to write five things that make me special:

I am a good listener.

I am smart and am always searching for new knowledge in order to expand my perceptions.

I am a good hugger.

I am a genuine person with a soft heart.

I am courageous and strong. I can endure anything with God in my life.

I feel better already!

Friday, August 16, 1998

   I am tired tonight so I'll be brief.

I am grateful for a nice day spent with my cousin, Amanda I enjoyed the company and conversation.

I am grateful (for) my loving family.

I am grateful for the energy I still have.

I am grateful for my comfy bed.

I am grateful for my conversation with my special grandma. She is truly a blessing.

Sunday, August 18, 1998

   Today I feel blessed to be alive and doing as well as I am. I went to see Elena today and it was a very difficult visit. She is beginning to lose that sparkle in her eyes and her body is starting to give up. As I was leaving, Greg took me aside and asked me to think about ideas for her memorial service. I really wasn't ready for that. I guess I've been in denial that "it" was really going to happen.. I just keep hoping for a miracle and today Greg's words hit me like a ton of bricks! Elena is so special to me. We've been fighting our battles along side each other for the past four years. Her strength and courage were what kept me going many times. It scares me to think that she may soon be gone.

   After today's events I really feel lucky to feel as good as I do. I feel lucky to Have lived the 22 years that I have.

   Also today I was fortunate enough to start another semester at Hancock and for this I am grateful. (I'll finish college sooner or later.)

   I was then set up on a double date by Bridgett and Matt. I am grateful for my baby sister who knows how lonely I am sometimes. She helped to bring back hope of finding love and feeling like I deserve.

Overall, today was a busy day filled with a variety of emotions, but I am happy to be alive.

Thursday, September 10, 1998

    It has been a while since I last wrote my gratitude list. Elena's passing has really overwhelmed me and I just haven't felt like writing.

    Today I am grateful for the beautiful sunshine.

    I thank God for blessing me with the time I got to spend with Elena and for the closeness that formed between our families.

    I am grateful to have a wonderful grandma who I have planned a trip to see.

    I am thankful for my loving family.

I am grateful for a fulfilling day in which I got a lot accomplished.

    I am thankful for the energy that flowed through me which allowed me to get things done.

    I am thankful for a beautiful day filled with sunshine.

    I am thankful for God's little blessings that make our earth enjoyable.

    I'm grateful for my improving sense of well being.

Chapter Thirteen

<u>A visit with Grandma Verna</u>

Monday, September 28, 1998

I finally made it to grandma's house and I am so grateful to be here. I can think of millions of things to list on my gratitude list that all pertain to her. She is so wise and gives me unconditional love. I feel so safe when I'm with her. A couple of nights ago we sat out on her porch swing and we talked. She reminisced about her childhood. I could almost see the house she grew up in: "Fairview."

Sadly she recalls how things changed when the depression hit. Her father tried to hold on to "Fairview" for about 3 years, but had to keep selling things, including her horse. She doesn't talk more about what life turned into, only that things were really hard.

They moved to Chicago (the city) and Fairview was forever a memory. I can't imagine going from having everything to having nothing. You can see the sadness in grandma's eyes, so she stops talking about it and changes the subject. I am so grateful for that conversation.

Tuesday, September 29, 1998

Today is my last day at grandmas. Last night I cried at the thought of having to return to my roller coaster life at home. Gram crawled into bed with me and cuddled. She told me that she is always with me even though her physical body isn't and that I will always be her "baby girl." I cried more. She told me about memories of her and Marie to help me not to think about leaving. About how they raided a garden patch after walking home from Joey Kolenowski's and ate so much cabbage they got sick (especially when they returned home to find her Mom cooking sauerkraut.

She also told me about their first smoking experience when she was about 11. They found some of her Dad's old cigars and went down to the basement. Her Mom caught them and when Father returned home to find 2 "green" girls he offered that they all smoke a cigarette. The thought made both of them sick to their stomachs. That was punishment enough. Gram and Marie sure were mischievous!

What a lady! She is such a survivor. Lucky for me I have her genes floating around in me.

Chapter Fourteen

Angst

Monday, December 28, 1998

I am slowly sinking into a pit of depression. I can't remember the last time I felt good. Things seem to keep going wrong and I fear that my mental state is causing them to happen. I struggle to hold on to hope and not give up. It pains me even to think of the result. Death haunts me and invades my mind often. Part of me believes it would be the easiest way, but I don't want to give up. I need for something to go right so my hope will be restored. Just for once to feel that I am taking a step forward instead of backsliding. Tonight I feel so over-whelmed and I wish I could scream. No one understands what it is like to be me!!! No one knows how uncomfortable it feels to be inside my body…the pain, the itching, the blurred vision, the shortness of breath, the wheezing, I could go on. I don't remember what it felt like to be healthy and I am having a hard time envisioning myself of getting there again.

Chapter Fifteen

<u>In darkness springs hope</u>

Thursday, December 31, 1998

The last day of 1998—what a year it has been. Supposed to be the year of the cure, but it just didn't happen. I can't say that it was better/worse, it just was. What I shall try to remember is the progress made and not the backsliding, the happy moments, not the sad. Although it comes to mind that we lost our special baby, Elena, and that is hard not to be sad about. We also had the birth of Austin to my niece Christy and Jim, and that was happy.

Ongoing chemotherapy treatments, radiation on Amber's L3 vertebrate, and pneumonia speckled the year. Yet I feel a gift of closeness that Amber and I have truly come to know with each other. The excitement of getting ready to go on our fabulous family cruise on the HMS Holiday to Catalina Island and Ensenada, and the great time we had with each other was a highlight. All these things and many more I am not accounting for.

The year was a mix of emotions and an escalating need for help outside our family unit from therapists, sponsors, nurses and our extended community church family in prayer. I can't say we were left alone to fend for ourselves. The Macedo's, even in their time of grief and loss, have continually been support for us. My sisterhood with

Julie is a blessing to me.

The tragedy of death, the fear of dying and being left behind, the absolute terror of loss has been unmistakable this year. I vow to begin the new year with new hope and a fresh outlook on some new possibilities 1999 will be a better year.

Elena
Sparkling eyes of blue
Curly blonde locks so soft
A hug that warms your insides
A giggle that warms your heart

Imagination without boundaries
Art that makes you smile
Innocence that's overwhelming
Purity of soul admired by all

Close friend and play companion
A soul mate sent from God
Smiles that warmed my spirit
That carried me through it all

Her journey was not easy
Too young to endure such pain
Yet able to seize the moment
And live the most each day

Unfair that she had to leave me
This gift sent from up above
Her memory will always be with me
And remembered most with her family's love

We will meet again someday
Our souls will be united
Till then she will guide and protect me
Send me smiles, be by my side

Amber Carter

Chapter Sixteen

The Light Begins to Fade

Tuesday, January 19, 1999

When the New Year celebrating has worn off, the inevitable daily pains of life take hold. Despite my overwhelming feeling of fear and despair, I am determined to forge ahead and create a façade of hope, security, and wellness. These last two days have been so very hard. Amber has developed shingles again. This poor child of mine, dear to my heart and brave to the core, has suffered yet one more indignity. She is trying to maintain some control in her life, but one thing after another is zapping her ability to call any of her own shots.

The current chemotherapy drug is presenting the biggest problem. That which is supposed to save her from the evils of cancer is just becoming a subtle enemy. It is like she is stuck between two evils pulling at her weakened body, creating a mental and physical hurdle she is not equipped to clear. No longer able to tolerate anti-depressants due to heart fibrillations, she is left with battling depression some other way. It is hard not to be down when you feel your body is out of control and life is passing you by.

I am scared—really scared for the first time. I'm not alone in my fear. Bridgett broke down last night after watching her sissy try to keep down her dinner and finally succumbing to dry heaves instead.

Somehow I feel responsible to divert my family from the pain we are all going through. God help me to have the strength and imagination to do this and keep my family surviving as a unit.

Tuesday, January 19, 1999
The eventual visit to Dr. Dan happened. The reading of the C.A.T. scans, now a firm family ritual, came to pass. As he placed each picture on the lighted shelf, one slice to the next of Amber's neck and chest, my heart sank with each one. We had all been taking our moods from Amber, and as she sat pensively, didn't flinch. She took the news as bravely as Joan of Arc at the stake. The divine wisdom of her knowledge was flowing out from her onto us. Her silent smile and poignant acceptance fate handed to her was amazing. Amazing Grace.
The disease had not made its exit out of her lungs and was stubbornly planting new seeds there.

Friday, February 12, 1999
Warm sunshine on my face as I sit outside in the back yard. I feel direction less. I'm not quite sure what I want or should be doing. My head is cloudy today and I feel as though I'm half asleep. I zone out, not really thinking of anything. I guess my body just needs to "BE," my minds the one fighting its inclination. Then I start to feel guilty because I'm being lazy.
  —soft breeze across my face tickling my ears
  —light sound and birds conversing with each other, so much to say
  —cat's cleaning himself wants some attention
I would like to come back as a cat. A soft orange cat like Milo…a lover but full of spunk. Always part kitten with infinite curiosity.
Someone's listening to Riverdance, I can hear it. must be the neighbor a few houses up the street. I know it's not "neighbor boy." At least the music is pleasant.
I long for Spring. Today almost feels like it, but the breeze is still cold.

Wednesday, April 14, 1999
My dreams have left me with thoughts I don't want to have. Dying.
I wrote it in my dream, I was crying, had gone shopping for groceries, and written down dying on my list.
Yesterday I spent the entire morning calling about a clinical trial involving positive Epstein-Barr virus patients at Baylor University Hospital in Texas. Amber had been tested positive for it and having had a BMT already and relapsed she definitely qualified for participating in the trial. Dr. Heslop is head researcher and I had done some e-mail-

ing to her, but this was the first time I had heard her voice. Excited to share the information with Amber, I was in the middle of speaking to the doctor when Amber got up out of bed. I acted as if I were planning her wedding No doubt I overwhelmed her and it set the stage for the rest of the morning being filled with fear and worry about doing the "right thing."

There was so much to do if we were going to get in on the trial. Bone marrow and blood samples had to be Fed Exed to the hospital ASAP. But Amber was slipping away inch by inch, mentally and physically. It was becoming too much, and I didn't know how far to push anymore. She used to be right beside me, searching for new treatments, printing information from the computer. Now I was taking that seat. How could I keep instilling hope in her?

Friday, April 16, 1999
> *Frustrated*
> *Itchy*
> *Like I'm disappointing everyone.*
> *Scared*
> *Like I'm going crazy*
> *Sorry*
> *Sad*
> *Alone (no one has a clue what its like to be me)*

Friday, April 16, 1999

Last night Amber and I went to our weekly watercolor class. I had found that painting was something we could do to feel creative and it didn't take much physical energy. Having had chemo that morning, I was uncertain she would want to go, but she still did. She had been working on a boat with a single fisherman in it. Using her favorite shades of green, she mastered the art of reflection on the lake perfectly. Her teacher, Roseanne, commented on its beauty and simplicity, that Amber had captured true isolation. Little did her teacher know, she had become a pro at it from personal experience.

When her piece was put up for the class to see, I could feel the suspense, but she was rock solid in her rendition of a mere photo found in National Geographic picked up at the doctor's office. The class's response went from, "good composition," to "great value range." Her self-confidence soaring, she accepted the compliments with aplomb. It was indeed a shining moment for her.

Chapter Seventeen

<u>Retreat</u>

Saturday, April 24, 1999
Women's Retreat with Julie

    I was drawn to the swing set. I want so much to be a kid again, when I was so innocent and pure. Free of worries and fear, everything was so new and fascinating. To swing was like flying and I could do it for hours. I didn't worry about being productive or about meeting societies' expectations. I could just be. Made me think of Elena. I miss her!

    While on the swing I noticed a rock sitting all by itself just waiting to be discovered. Hidden under the dust were beautiful specks of color. The rock was smooth as I picked it up and it fit into the palm of my hand. I was meant to find it. In many ways I would like to be a rock. My life feels like it is falling apart and I would like to feel solid and whole again.

    I also desire to have a faith that is as firm as this rock. Sometimes I feel so alone and I question whether or not God is listening.

    Along my path I spotted lavender, which is one of my favorite scents. The bloom represents peace, which I truly desire. My life seems so uncertain and I long for a sense of security and peace. Smelling the lavender gives me some comfort.

    I am amazed at the detail and miracle of nature. God created the most beautiful plants, flowers, sounds, smells. I could go on. What's more is that he blessed us with the senses that allow us to enjoy them. If only we took more time to listen, smell and feel all that is around us. Life is beautiful.

Monday, May 17, 1999

     Elena's birthday was two days ago and it has left me feeling empty and sad. She was such a special soul and it is so unfair that she wasn't allowed to stay here with those who loved her. I miss her smile and contagious giggle. She was so uplifting to be around despite all the junk she was going through. I admired her drive to do normal kid things even though she was going through adult stuff. She never seemed t feel sorry for herself. I wish I was more like her. I want to know what her secret was to being happy. Maybe it helps to be a kid.

     Ten things I'm grateful for today

The ability to hug and be hugged

The gift of compassion

Cats to cuddle with (especially Milo)

My Mom

My Dad

My sister

My good memory which safely stores special moments

Beautiful flowers that brighten my day

The Macedo Family who loves me and inspires me

The ability to see and hear all the beauty around me

Cambria 1999

My Darling Amber~
You are precious to me
    you are precious to my family
        and especially to Elena.

You share your love and joy,
    you share your beauty with my daughter
        a bandana, a choice to wear a smile
        and a laugh.

You played with her, understood her
    when understanding was hard
    and you brought her joy
        sometimes in a McDonald's toy
        sometimes in your hug and voice.

Your comfort at camp eased Elena's way
    gave grace to her and comforted her.,
        I cherish my pictures of you together.

And now, you live with memories and questions
    questions that are so big
        and bewildering to you
        and all of us.

Amber, you are so beautiful-
    never lose sight of this.
    your ways are to be respected
        and loved.
    your special needs to be cherished.

I know understanding is desired, but affirmation of you
    is what I want to give.

Allow grace to be in your life and good attempts
    (and near misses) and your friends...
        for we love you.

Julie Macedo

BOOK FIVE

NOWADAYS

Nowadays
Away from home
Up above
All I want to do
Is wish you well
Take care of mom
Love, Amber
~This is a good day~

Chapter One

<u>Who's to Blame, Anyway?</u>

In the very beginning of the illness, self-blame was abundant. She believed there was a flaw in her character, or a bad action, a lack of spirituality that resulted in the cancer being let loose in her body. I spent many a conversation assuring her that God was not punishing her for some misdeed. Even though I could not explain why, or how this evil encroached her being, I knew positively it was not due to anything she deserved for bad conduct of any kind.

The God I believe in these days is not of the punishing variety that I had known from my childhood. Instead I have cultivated one that could accept us as vulnerable, sinful, and intelligent human beings that are responsible for our own actions, good or bad, and yet love us anyway. And I refused to let her think for a minute she could have done anything large or small enough to receive a sentence of cancer.

After having read Rabbi Kushner's book, *Why Bad Things Happen to Good People* I try to come to an understanding. There is no answer. Just as the good doctor told us on our first visit, just quit asking the question and get on with ridding yourself of it. Unfortunately, the questions come back over and over again. Was it the pesticide used near the high school she attended? Was it the food I made for her as a baby? Maybe the well water she was raised on? Did she worry too much by going away to college, which allowed the immune system to malfunction? Is it in the family tree on her father's side? After all, we do not know her biological paternal grandfather's genetic make up. The "why" list goes on and on and on to infinity.

Kushner's explanation is that of a random evil present as the culprit. One is not chosen by God to be sacrificed, only chance, destiny, or fate, drop down and crap on one unlucky person regardless of race, age, gender or purity.

The boogey man would spread his wings and fly around her bedroom late in the evening after we had gone to bed. He would fill her head with self doubt, wreaking havoc with her serenity, and she would beckon me to come in and kiss her goodnight, and then keep me there with philosophical questions about life, plans for treatment, new ideas to try to keep her from going into the dark hole of depression. We would stay up deep into the night and I would try to soothe her by scratching her back, rubbing her legs and feet or even try reading to her. We began the <u>Great Gatsby</u> with high hopes of it being the first of many classics neither one of us had read.

My biblical friend, Donna, suggests by all she believes in that Amber had simply learned all that God had in mind. In her young life she had accumulated all the knowledge of goodness. Her job, as she went down the path God chose for her, was to touch people with that goodness and faith along the way. Simply put, to change people's lives with her gentle guidance. Donna was right; Amber never gave up on God. She stayed involved in the youth group at her church as long as she had the energy to do so. She believed in he, she, or it until the day she died and it gave her great comfort. But, so did love.

I often would tell her in times of fear and panic, "Do you believe in the power of love?" Through her tears she would look up at me and timidly say, "Yes." One of my most treasured possessions is a picture torn out of a Precious Moments coloring book. One day while she was alone she colored it with crayons, something she used to love to do as a small child. It was a little girl with her big blue eyes looking up and above her head Amber had written the words, "I believe in the Power of Love." Indeed.

Amberley

Flowing blonde hair
Growing past her
Slender shoulders

Sparkling blue eyes
Lids fringed with
Long brown lashes

A flawless, ivory complexion
Smoothly stretched over
An oval shaped bone structure

Cupid lips
Curtained over
White straight teeth

An ever-present smile
Outlined with perfection
And colored in
With New York City mauve

Delicate, petit, size 5
Curving in
Creating a well proportioned body
Dancers legs
Turned out at the hip

All ten toes painted
Pointed
Fragile
Sturdy
Stubborn
Loving
Lively
Courageous

Splendid hugs
Could wrap around your heart
And soul

Gentle touch
From well manicured fingers
That could reach beyond conversation
And send messages
To the stars and beyond

Intelligence groomed
Not flaunted
Not average
Such joy in learning
Perfection self-expected
Often attained

Fun loving
Friendly
Spiritual being
Intuitive heartstrings

Remembrance 2002
Janine

My Turn

And now
        My turn
        My test
        My sorrow
        My tears shall flow
Long past the 'morrow

The child I bore
        My love
        My source
        My dearest friend
On her own course

Her trip
        Alone
She shall be making

& I
        Alone
in grief
be taking

Janine Carter
7/9/99

AMBER LEAHANNE CARTER

August 8, 1976~June 10, 1999

Born in Albuquerque, New Mexico, Amber began dancing at the age of three. She danced in countless recitals and community gatherings to the delight of her family and friends. At the age of ten, she became a member of Danse Classique Theatre, a local ballet company in Albuquerque. While dancing with this company, she performed with the Bolshoi Ballet from Russia.

In 1989, Amber moved from New Mexico to the California Central Coast where she attended Judkins Middle School, and Arroyo Grande High School. She was a member of the Gilbert Reed Ballet from 1990~1992 and toured the public schools dancing in Peter and the Wolf as well as other productions. She became a cheerleader for AGHS in 1991, and also was a member of AGHS Dance Company all four years. Amber choreographed many numbers for Kaleidoscope and Dance Company in both ballet and jazz.

Amber graduated in the top of her class from AGHS in 1994, and was accepted to the University of San Diego, where she majored in Psychology. She attended school there until 1995, when she was diagnosed with Hodgkins Disease, a cancer of the lymph nodes. While undergoing chemotherapy and radiation, she continued her education at Allan Hancock College and continued to take ballet classes. She was placed on the Dean's Honor List for her outstanding academic performance while at Hancock.

Amber's fervent wish was to receive her Bachelor's Degree in Psychology so she could become a therapist and help others dealing with the struggles of having a life-threatening disease.

Her hobbies included watercolor painting, doing latch hook, and cuddling with her kitties and her family.

After an almost five-year battle with cancer, Amber passed away quietly at her home on June 10, 1999. She is remembered and loved by her family, Tom and Janine Carter and Bridgett Carter-Janowicz.

Memorial Service
Saint Patrick's Church

We wanted Amber's memorial service to be light hearted and unique so I asked a few special people to take some of her personal items up to the altar and say a few words to the congregation. We also had the band that usually played at the 6pm Sunday mass at St. Pat's play some selected songs, among them was a special song Jay Horn composed in memory of Amber, *Morning Glory*.

1.Toe Shoes (Bridgett)

Amber had a passion for dance. She was dancing before she was born. She began taking dance lessons from Miss Winnie at the age of 3 and when she was 10, Amber was ready for "pointe shoes." She danced in many studio productions in New Mexico, and some here in California with the Gilbert Reed Dance Company. Some of the best memories created were those of her sister, Bridgett and her Mom dancing to "Thank Heaven for Little Girls."

2.School Books (Krishanda)

Amber attended schools in both New Mexico and California, but her experiences and love of knowledge and the pursuit of it through studying and attending classes was universal. She did the usual "ditching to go to the beach" days, and her first and only semester at USD had her share of party times. When Amber was diagnosed with cancer, those days for school became much more goal oriented. Throughout chemotherapy, radiation, surgeries, bad hair days (no hair days) she was happiest when she got to complain about finals and projects that she had to finish.

3.Watercolor painting and beanie baby (Dr. Dan)

When Amber was no longer able to attend college, her quest for knowledge didn't stop there. She and her Mom took a watercolor class together. This painting was done at cancer camp with her favorite buddy, Dr. Dan.

4. Scarves ("Red")

When Amber lost her hair, she began to wear scarves. Her outfit was never complete without the perfect one. She took a great deal of pride in her appearance, and most people never knew she was "sick."

5. Camp shirts (Helen)

Camp Reach for the Stars was an annual pleasure for Amber and her family. Even though Amber was 18 at the time of diagnosis, she was still considered a kid with cancer to her young buddies at camp. There she met her most favorite kid, Elena Macedo.

Gentle thoughts and insights

ANGEL AMBER

Amber was my best friend. We shared so many passions in life; music, dancing, nature, hiking, the beach, and even the more simple things like boys and cookie dough ice cream. We understood each other and could tell what the other was thinking without having to speak, which we were both well aware of, and often joked about our "mental telepathy". We had a deep, loving connection and friendship. Amber was a true friend and a good listener. I could talk to her about anything and know she would understand and help me see things from a positive perspective. I remember going to her for advice for something so minor compared to the depth of her own challenges during her illness. Yet she still listened intently, smiled, and gave me the calming Amberley advice that she had always given so well. That is the kind of person Amber was, gentle, caring, compassionate and wise.

Amber loved to have a good time. If there were an opportunity for fun, Amber and I would go for it together. We would share the joy and good times and feed off of each other's happiness and later reminisce about all of our fond and silly memories with laughter. Because I know she would want me to think of all the good times we shared, that is how I like to remember Amber. Of course the sadness of her battle with cancer is always with me. I think of her every day of my life. But even though that sadness runs so deep, the happiness and love that I associate with Amber is so much greater.

Amber's graceful spirit has taught me so much about life's lessons. She has helped me to realize how extremely important it is to make time for the ones you love as you never know when that time will run out. Life can get so busy and crazy as we all know, but the times that we will really remember and cherish are those times we have spent together. When we are faced with losing someone so close and special, we will still have the memories and love, with their immortal power, to live on in our hearts and souls.

So realize how precious life is. Seize the day. Challenge yourself. Travel to new and exciting places. Learn about the world. Have compassion for others who are less fortunate than you without having pity. If you are having a hard day, just think of the friends, family, and loved ones in your life. Appreciate the simple things that surround us everywhere in nature. Enjoy the warmth of the sunshine, the sound of rushing water flowing down the river, the breeze whispering through the trees, the smell of the ocean, and the beauty of a blooming flower. All of these things remind me of Amber, as I know she took the time to appreciate them.

Amber was the kind of friend, the kind of person that only comes around once in a life-time. I am so fortunate to have shared a part of my life in her company.

With loving memories,
Krishanda Joy Struble

Dear Carter Family,
It is so hard to say goodbye to Amber. She was so kind so sweet and so full of love…
She loved her family
She loved cats and angels and dance—
And she loved me.
She was so easy to spend time with
Such a joy to spend time with

God may have taken Amber away from us—
but he will never take away the beautiful
memories that she left with us.

What a smile. It would just light you up.

You are a great family.
Best wishes,

Love always,
Dr. D.

To my friend Janine, who has shared more of her life with me than she probably ever planned, I thank you for your courage and tenacity in sharing your love story of your daughter Amber. In this story I can see, feel, and hear you and Amber continuing to talk and love each other and it has given me a beautiful glimpse of heaven.

Your friend forever, Marilyn

Prologue

Amber lived the most fundamental truths in life. She had courage, the strength to venture and withstand danger, fear and difficulty.

Through courage one is able to find trust, a reliance on character, strength and truth.

Through trust is found hope and a desire for obtainment of expectations, which then allows more courage.

To persevere is not easy; to do gracefully is an art.

Amber knew art.

Amber, like a beautiful swan gliding on a reflective lake, was a beautiful example of courage.

Ann Fontenou "Red"

Dear Amber,

Wasn't it just yesterday we were praying together? Wow, what a privilege to have been praying with you, Amber. It isn't often I get the opportunity to sit and pray with young people. Everyone's in a hurry, including me. But you calmed me, as hard as that is to believe. We talked about your latest treatment or the last treatment that wasn't working. You never showed signs of discouragement. You knew there was something out there that would work. I'd leave making deals with God, saying, "Lord, make this treatment work. Give her that much deserved miracle." Every morning praying, pleading with god, saying, "Lord, she's your beautiful child, yes, but she belongs here with her family and the people whose lives she's touched." We needed her here. We needed her courage. We needed her sweet, gentle spirit.

I remember at the Ecumenical service a couple years ago, they passed the cross around. I thought, she's so short. Everyone around was taller than us. You couldn't quite reach the cross, poor kid. I took your arm and reached it up. There, I thought, put that awful disease on His cross. There, that's better.

And you kept fighting the good fight. Never showing signs of discouragement. Was that bravery for my benefit? It worked. I'd go home thinking anything I had stressed about earlier in the day was insignificant compared to your struggle. So did God put you in my life as a gift? Yes, I believe so. I learned compassion, perseverance, patience and joy from you. You taught me what having a quiet courage is really all about.

How did I come to know Amber? At first, Amber was just a name on a prayer list. Then one of my daughters put a face on the name. "You remember her, Mom," she said, "The little girl from youth group. She's a year ahead of Leah at school." I became heavy-hearted that such a pretty little one could be so sick. Soon after I started to make notes to myself to remember to pray for her. Then one Sunday I introduced myself to her, saying, "Just wanted you to know someone was praying for you." Renew started and I asked if you would help. You didn't even hesitate. Did anyone know but me that you were going through treatment while facilitating a group of youth through six weeks of faith sharing? Did anyone know you typed the program every week before the following week? Never a complaint about how unorganized we were. And what a success that first season was. We couldn't have done it without you.

I guess it sounds like I'm making you out to sound like a saint. I only saw your goodness. Well, I can go on and on, but I want to say it was an honor to be one of your prayer warriors. Now you can pray for us. I'll thank God once more for putting you in my life. You were truly a flower. Now you know the true meaning of God's peace and glory. Go with God, Amber. Like the song, will you remember us? We will remember you. I will remember you always with love.

Sharon Brandy

Epilogue

Angels are everywhere. They are all around us, helping us, protecting us, guiding us. Once in a while, we are lucky and get to know one. I knew one. You have met her in the pages of this book. Let her story change your life, as it did mine

Although she wasn't a saint, or perfect, she was an angel. She was you, me, our daughter, our son, our mother, our sister, our friend – our friend's daughter. She was a teenager trying to get on with the business of living – choreographing her future.

Although she had every reason to rail against the heavens, feel sorry for herself every day of her struggle with cancer; cash it all in, she chose instead to live with grace, fortitude, hope and humility. She taught us these things and more. She tutored us in Life 101.

Amber Carter died on June 10, 1999, at the age of twenty-two, but her future lives on. Her journey, though brief, was vital. She modeled how to live. She humiliated death. She taught us to be humane, but more importantly, she taught us how to love. She continues to teach and to touch. She survives in the love and courage she gifted to those whose lives she touched.

She was a hero, because a hero isn't necessarily brave; a hero quietly does what has to be done. But she was brave. One of the bravest women I will ever know, aside from her mother.

Janine Carter and all the moms of the world who stand by helplessly watching their child suffer should never have to do just that. Dad's shouldn't have to flail at windmills they can never conquer, trying to protect their families. Sisters should fight, laugh, love one another without feeling there just isn't enough time – because there never is.

The Carter's of the world are our friends, our neighbors; they are us. Their story is about mankind as one big family. We need to take better care of each other. We need to help shoulder burdens.

Children should never die before their parents, it upsets the order, is cruel beyond endurance. Yet through the example Amber set for her family, they survived and will continue to survive and thrive. Through Amber's legacy of love, they make a difference on this planet. They, too, are angels. Every single day, they take their pain and turn it into soothing balms. Amber's love of life is unleashed through her nephews. Amber dances with every recipient of the Amber Carter Scholarship. Her long legs run alongside her mom at every cancer run fundraiser. And Amber helps Mom, Dad and Bridgett soothe, grieve, and help others who have to travel the roads they traveled as a family

Amber's angel message lives on through everyone who reads her story and will think about, maybe pray for, but definitely visit the neighbor down the street, the cousin, Grandmother, or stranger battling disease, loneliness, alienation. Cancer eats the body; friendship and love nourish the soul.

Amber's angel message is love.

Suzanne Caplette-Champeau

Medical treatment timeline chart (1995–1997). Rows are organized by treatment category, each subdivided into WEEKS 1–4. Columns are months (J F M A M J J A S O N D) for each year. Filled dots (•) indicate occurrences.

Treatment	Weeks	1995 — J F M A M J J A S O N D	1996 — J F M A M J J A S O N D	1997 — J F M A M J J A S O N D
Procedures / Tests	1	• •	· · • • · · · · · · · ·	· · · · · · · · · · • ·
	2	•	· • · · · · • · · · · ·	
	3	• •	• · • • · · • · · · · ·	
	4	• •	• • • · · · • · · · · ·	
Surgery	1			•
	2		· · · · · · • · · · · ·	
	3	· •		
	4	•		
Chemo	1	· · • • • • • • • • • ·	· · · · • • · · · · · ·	• • · · · · · · • · · • •
	2	· · • • • · · · · • · •	· · · · • · · · · · · ·	· · · · • · · · • •• · •
	3	· · · • · · · · · · · ·		· · · · · · · · · · · •
	4	· · · · • • • · · · · ·		· • · · · · · · •• · • •
Radiation	1		· • •• · · · · ••• · ·	
	2		· • •• · · · · ••• · ·	
	3		· • •• · · · · ••• · ·	
	4		· • •• · · · · ••• · ·	
C.A.T. Scan / X-Ray	1	· •	· • • · · · · · · · · ·	• • • • · · · · · · · ·
	2	· · · · · · · · · • · ·	· • · · · · · · · · · ·	· · · · · · · · • · · ·
	3	· · · · · · · • · · · ·	• • • · · · · · · · · ·	· · · · · · · · • · • ·
	4	· • · · · • · · · · · ·	• • · · · · · · · · · ·	
Transfusion	1		· · • · · · · · · · · ·	
	2		· · • · · · · · · · · ·	· • · · · · · · · · · ·
	3		· • • · · · · · · · · ·	· • · • · · · · · · · ·
	4			• · · · · · · • · • • •
CBC	1	· • • • • • • • • • • ·	· · • · · • · · · • · ·	· · • • · · · • • • • •
	2	• • • • • • • • • • · •	· · • · • · · • • · · ·	• • · · • • • · · · • •
	3	• • • • • • • • • • • ·	· · · · · · · • · · · ·	• • · · • • • • · · • ·
	4	· • • • • • · · • · · ·	• · · · · · · · • · · ·	• · • · · • • · · · ••
Procrit Injections	1		· ••• · · · · · · · · ·	
	2		· ••• · · · · · · · · ·	
	3		· ••• · · · · · · · · ·	
	4		· ••• · · · · · · · · ·	
Apherisis Stem Cells	1		· •• • · · · · · · · · ·	
	2		· •• · · · · · · · · · ·	
	3		· • · · · · · · · · · ·	
	4		· • · · · · · · · · · ·	

Vertical label in the 1996 column (spanning the Procedures/Tests and Surgery rows): **TRANSPLANT**

	WEEKS	1998 J	F	M	A	M	J	J	A	S	O	N	D	1999 J	F	M	A	M	J	J	A	S	O	N	D
Procedures / Tests	1						•		•																
	2																								
	3	•						•																	
	4							•																	
Surgery	1																								
	2																								
	3																								
	4																								
Chemo	1	•	•	•	•			•	•		•		•				•	•	•						
	2		•	•		•	•				•		•				•	•							
	3	•		•			•	•		•	•	•	•		•	•	•								
	4		•			•	•						•			•		•							
Radiation	1						•	•	•																
	2						•																		
	3						•																		
	4						•																		
C.A.T. Scan / X-Ray	1	•						•			•	•		•											
	2			•				•							•										
	3						•	•					•	•											
	4							•						•		•									
Transfusion	1				•				•					•		•		•							
	2													•		•		•							
	3									•	•				•										
	4	•						•								•									
CBC	1	•	•	•	•	•	•	•	•	•	•	•	•	•	•	•	•	•	•						
	2	•	•	•	•	•	•	•	•	•	•	•	•	•	•	•	•	•	•						
	3	•	•	•	•	•	•	•	•	•	•	•	•	•	•	•	•	•	•						
	4	•	•	•	•	•	•	•	•	•	•	•	•	•	•	•	•	•							
Procrit Injections	1																								
	2																								
	3																								
	4																								
Apherisis Stem Cells	1																								
	2																								
	3																								
	4																								